SILENCE AND SEIZURE

Life Writing Series

Wilfrid Laurier University Press's Life Writing series celebrates life writing as both genre and critical practice. As a home for innovative scholarship in theory and critical practice, the series embraces a range of theoretical and methodological approaches, from literary criticism and theory to autoethnography and beyond, and encourages intersectional approaches attentive to the complex interrelationships between gender, class, race, ethnicity, sexuality, ability, and more. In its commitment to life writing as genre, the series incorporates a range of life writing practices and welcomes creative scholarship and hybrid forms. The Life Writing series recognizes the diversity of languages, and the effects of such languages on life writing practices within the Canadian context, including the languages of migration and translation. As such, the series invites contributions from voices and communities who have been under- or misrepresented in scholarly work.

SILENCE

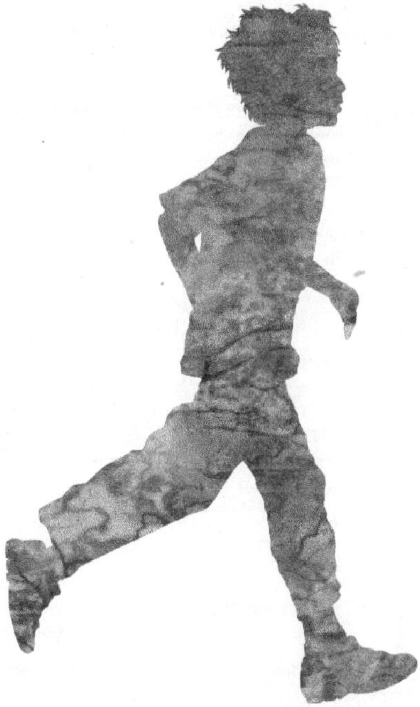

& SEIZURE

Parenting Through Complexity

CHRISTINE STEWART-NUÑEZ

WILFRID LAURIER UNIVERSITY PRESS

Wilfrid Laurier University Press acknowledges the support of the Canada Council for the Arts for our publishing program. We acknowledge the financial support of the Government of Canada through the Canada Book Fund for our publishing activities. Funding provided by the Government of Ontario and the Ontario Arts Council. This work was supported by the Research Support Fund.

Library and Archives Canada Cataloguing in Publication

Title: Silence and seizure : parenting through complexity / Christine Stewart-Nuñez.
Names: Stewart-Nuñez, Christine, author
Series: Life writing series.
Description: Series statement: Life writing series | Includes bibliographical references and index.
Identifiers: Canadiana (print) 20260106275 | Canadiana (ebook) 20260106291 | ISBN 9781771127332 (softcover) | ISBN 9781771127363 (PDF) | ISBN 9781771127356 (EPUB)
Subjects: LCSH: Stewart-Nuñez, Christine—Family. | LCSH: Parents—United States—Biography. | LCSH: Epileptic children—United States—Biography. | LCSH: Parenting—United States. | LCGFT: Autobiographies.
Classification: LCC RJ496.E6 S74 2026 | DDC 362.19892/8360092—dc23

Cover and interior design: Michel Vrana. Copy editor: Julie McGonegal.

Waterloo, Ontario, Canada
www.wlupress.wlu.ca

This book is printed on FSC® certified paper. It contains recycled materials and other controlled sources, is processed chlorine-free, and is manufactured using biogas energy.
Printed in Canada

MIX
Paper | Supporting responsible forestry
FSC® C103567

CERTIFIED CANADIAN PUBLISHER

Wilfrid Laurier University Press is located on the Haldimand Tract, part of the traditional territories of the Haudenosaunee, Anishinaabe, and Neutral Peoples. This land is part of the Dish with One Spoon Treaty between the Haudenosaunee and Anishinaabe Peoples and symbolizes the agreement to share, to protect our resources, and not to engage in conflict. We are grateful to the Indigenous Peoples who continue to care for and remain interconnected with this land. Through the work we publish in partnership with our authors, we seek to honour our local and larger community relationships, and to engage with the diversity of collective knowledge integral to responsible scholarly and cultural exchange.

I dedicate this book to my parents,
my first teachers of unconditional love
and to my children,
who continue to nurture those lessons.

TABLE OF CONTENTS

Preface

INTER: prefix noting between

FOR MEMOIRISTS, THE METHODS BY WHICH WE DECIDE HOW to represent our characters vary.[1] Whether or not the people we depict consent to their inclusion in our writing adds tension to the method selection. Sometimes writers seek permission. Sometimes characters offer feedback and the writer alters the scene. Sometimes names are changed or identifying details obscured. Sometimes characters are deleted, leaving a ghost presence in a scene. I've used all of these methods in this book. But the decision about which method to choose becomes more complex when a parent writes about their own child—especially when that child is intellectually or cognitively disabled.

When I first began publishing poems that engaged with my son's seizure disorder, getting Holden's consent to share details about him would have been impossible. Despite poems holding no allegiance to veracity—I could hide behind the author/speaker separation—I still made decisions about what to include and exclude with great care, knowing that many readers would assume the poems were true.[2] I wanted to honour the authenticity at the heart of my work, so I centred my interpretations of Holden's seizure disorder, focusing on my observations as his mother. I didn't claim to tell his story. I didn't claim to know his thoughts or feelings.

When I began to publish creative nonfiction essays in which Holden appeared as a character, I researched ethical approaches to writing about one's children—and one's disabled children in particular. Essays require a more robust honesty.[3] The author is the narrator; the author claims the "I." Even if memories blur at the edges, essays require emotional truth, intentional truth. I developed a specific approach to represent my neurodivergent child in my essays.

First, I confronted the question of privacy. In stating facts about Holden's seizure disorder, was I betraying his privacy? Holden's seizure disorder could not be kept private since its effects could be seen at home, at school, and in our community. I considered how dangerous it could be for others to misinterpret Holden's behaviour; keeping the reasons secret might increase that risk. Keeping it private might also reinforce the stigma and myths that circulate around epilepsy. Fear and misinformation can prove fatal. I wanted readers to know more about epilepsy than I did at the beginning.

Second, I analyzed my motivation for writing. Why did I feel compelled to tell these stories? In memoir, writers grapple with life's tensions to gain insight; they publish stories about their own lives so that others might see possibilities, too. This wrestling motivated my practice before I became a mother, and it only deepened after I became a mother to a chronically ill and disabled child. It may not be the best or most complete answer, but it's the one that remains the most consistent. The insights generated through writing have sustained me and invited me to become a better mother, a better partner, a better human. I remind myself of this truth when writing gets hard to do.

Third, I tried to hold myself accountable to emotional honesty by asking if I would want someone writing about me in the ways I wrote about Holden. Both Holden and I have experienced vulnerability. Both of us know our body's betrayal—his through errant neuronal activity, mine through miscarriage. I aimed to represent Holden as the full, complex human being he is, subject to a range of emotions, and I leaned into my own embodied experiences, revealing moments when I grappled with my flaws, my anger, and my insufficiencies.

When I began to write a full-length memoir, privacy, motivation, and representation weren't enough. I thought more deeply about the impact of my writing on Holden and with my engagement with disability writ large. I found it difficult to ascertain the potential impact on Holden's feelings since he might not understand if I asked directly. Indirect ways surfaced. I noticed that when I recorded a video of him struggling with a task, such as reading, he'd want to see it again and again, but it distressed him to show the neuropsychologist, for whom I'd recorded the video. However, when I took a photo of him making progress, such as using an abacus to add and subtract, he'd want to see it again and again and want me to show *everyone*. I interpreted his reluctance to show the neuropsychologist videos of his struggle as feeling bad about his emotional response. Later on, I observed that his anxiety would surface if he thought that he—or even someone in the room or on a screen—wasn't making good choices. He always seemed to take pride in sharing his good work and his good behaviour. Now it doesn't distress him to talk about difficult moments from the past, and he still enjoys sharing his accomplishments.

I also began to study disability theory and activist practices.[4] These works increased my awareness of how to confront stereotypes that circulate about disabled bodies. With more care, I deepened my attempts to resist or revise disability tropes: the grief process of diagnosis, the fixing/curing trajectory, the viewpoint that locates the problem of disability in the disabled body. In doing so, I hope to decrease the stigma assigned to disability and add to conversations about what it means to reorient one's life as a parent of a disabled child.

The years I spent revising this memoir paralleled the resolution of Holden's seizure disorder and the expansion of his facility with language. Consequently, my approach to consent evolved even further. From time to time, I would describe a scene or moment from the manuscript and ask him if I could share it with others—if I could include it in my book—and he always said yes. Sometimes when he saw me at my laptop, he'd ask, "Are you writing about me?" with a big smile on his face. When I encountered Hannah Quinn and Rebecca-Eli Long's "Consent-as-Method: Capacity to Consent of Cognitively Disabled People and Research Ethics Review," I learned a better language for my approach: "Research is a relationship" and "Capacity is felt and done together."[5] They argue, "Consent-as-method is about actively creating ways to apply the felt knowledge of coercion and cultivate space for good feelings around consent."[6]

One of the ways I cultivated space for good feelings around consent was by reading the manuscript aloud with Holden present. I edited *Silence and Seizure* in my dining room while Holden played video games nearby. From time to time, he asked, "When did that happen?" or commented on a detail he remembered. Another way included going over photos and videos of events the memoir referenced. Because visual literacy is one of Holden's strengths, and because images often elicit the strongest responses from him, we looked through his scrapbooks together. When a set of photos corresponded with a passage from *Silence and Seizure*, we discussed his feelings about those scenes and about sharing those stories. When I pointed to one photo of him struggling through a meltdown, he said, "I'm not like that anymore." As we conversed, I realized just how true that is—just how much this book doesn't represent who Holden is today. When I asked him, "What would you like readers to know about nineteen-year-old Holden?" he replied, "That I'm a good person, and I feel a whole lot better."

This memoir is a project of literary becoming. It covers a period when I was grappling with how to adapt to the chaotic, identity-challenging changes in my life. Holden and I were both in process; we still are. Perhaps that is, for now, my strongest insight about my experiences. We are always becoming, and we should prioritize that becoming.

Once, I wondered if Holden would ever be able to read the words I wrote. Once, I wondered whether I'd ever be able to tell this story. Now I dream that he'll create his own narratives—through words or photography or art or cooking, whatever mediums bring him joy and laughter. My hopes for both my child and this book feel parallel in yet another way: to watch them do good work in the world and contribute to its flourishing.

Prologue

INTERSECTION: a cutting between

WHEN MY SON HOLDEN WAS THREE AND A HALF, HIS DAD, ABEL, and I took him to Krakow, Prague, and Munich. I'd been co-leading a study-abroad trip in Poland, and my family joined me for a vacation when my university students returned home. The trip highlighted Holden's gregarious personality and creativity.

One evening in Munich, as we stuffed ourselves with pretzels and *spaetzle*, Holden described the monsters he made from sticker books and chatted as he traced his own hand with different crayons to make turkeys, peacocks, and fish. As the conversation among the adults lingered, he looked out the restaurant's windows and spied a group of boys kicking around a soccer ball in a park. He yanked on my hand, leading me out of the restaurant.

"I want to play, too!" He pointed to them. "Please?" We took a few steps closer. The boys, several years older, spoke English and welcomed him. I watched my brown-haired boy chase the ball around the field as fast as his legs could carry him. His courage pleased me, although it wasn't new. Holden loved to organize play with his preschool friends by inviting them to build with blocks, look at books, or play with cars.

"Watch me kick the ball!" Holden said. "Look! I did it!" Amused by his play-by-play, his new friends laughed. We let him play until dusk pulled us back toward our hotel.

Travelling focused my attention; I learned so much about Holden on that trip. I relished his curiosity and spontaneity. Touring a medieval castle in Krakow, he ran across the tiered arcade, then zigzagged in and out of exhibits of coronation swords and armour. In restaurants, he sampled pork cutlets, fried cauliflower, roasted chicken, and fresh greens—pierogis and orange-glazed crepes his favourites. He commented on the languages spoken around him, noting how different they sounded from his own. In Prague, he celebrated modes of transportation new to him: horse-drawn carts, supersized escalators, and city buses. He stepped off the subway platform as if he'd conquered the moon. I felt as if I'd conquered something too, experiencing my passions—travelling and learning—with my child.

* * *

Three years later, when Holden was six and a half, our summer vacation was radically different. Abel and I had divorced. Holden had been diagnosed with epilepsy. My grand sightseeing tour was now limited to the other side of the state I lived in—South Dakota—where we joined a friend from high school and his family.

For the first two hours on Interstate 90, Holden stared ahead in the van while the other kids played their handheld video games. I'd hoped the other boys would spark some connection, perhaps even play. I expected laughter. Some fart jokes. Maybe even a squabble or two. But Holden just zoned out.

When we arrived at the Badlands and found a place to picnic, Holden seemed antsy as we ate our sandwiches. He didn't want to get back into the car to drive through the national park, but when we stopped at a scenic spot to take photos, he refused to get out. As I stood there trying to decide how to persuade him, he suddenly jumped out of the car and sprinted toward a steep slope, nearly tripping over the sign that read, "No foot traffic beyond this point." At Mount Rushmore, I posed for photographs with my friend's family, but Holden sat cross-legged, chin resting in his palm, eyes drooping in boredom. Even when one of the boys challenged Holden to a race, he meandered at a snail's pace. Halfway around the loop circling the monument, Holden sat down on the path. Tourists flowed around him. He wouldn't move until my friend offered him a piggyback ride to the car.

On that trip, I collected more worrisome moments: Holden urinated in his car seat midway across the state, even though he'd been using the toilet by himself for years—even though I'd just asked him if he needed to go. And he did it again, just a few miles from our destination. That time he'd told me he had to go, but not with enough notice to find a gas station. As I stripped the lining from his booster seat, replaced it with a towel, and dug out another set of fresh clothes from his suitcase, I watched him watching me. He seemed confused.

The next night, Holden fixated on controlling a game of putt-putt golf, unwilling to take turns or follow the rules. He ploughed through each segment by launching the golf ball any which way. Then he crashed out cold on the bed before dinner—and well before his usual bedtime. I remember telling my friend that I wasn't sure what I was going to do about Holden; inside, I didn't think I had the skills to confront what I was observing in my son—something difficult, something perplexing.

* * *

Once, I thought articulating how a child could change so much in just three years would be the story to tell; now I understand the story to be how I shifted from being the mother of a typically developing, healthy child to the mother of one with a chronic health condition and disability.[1]

When I look back at the South Dakota trip, the liminal space I occupied reveals itself. I knew something else was happening with Holden beyond the kinds of seizures medical professionals described; his struggles with words, sleep, and play meant something more, but I couldn't yet name it. Our world had shifted profoundly, yet I still wanted to measure our lives by the usual tools: vacations, sightseeing, picnics, putt-putt golf. In hindsight, I see how I inhabited a place where the medical model of disability and the social model of disability overlapped.[2] I understood Holden's seizures and wanted medication to stop them, but I didn't yet understand how my lack of words and frameworks created a barrier that disabled Holden just as much as the seizures did. I applied the pressures of what I thought our family should do because that's what seemed normal; in reality, neither of us needed normal.

That's the insidious nature of ableism, which assumes disabled people require fixing, frames difference as defect, and classifies disabled people as "less than."[3] It filters our expectations without our even knowing. It shapes our actions without our even feeling the pressure. Its frequency is so far outside our range that we don't feel its presence—until something tunes our perception and then we recognize how it saturates our laws, schools, languages, environments, and attitudes. Ableism is omnipresent, and its omnipresence is oppressive.

It's painful for me to admit how long it took me to locate disability, to touch its textured edges. It's embarrassing to recall that summer and how, even after all the evidence that Holden was changing, I didn't consider that I needed to change too. Regret haunts me. Did disability carry so much stigma that it didn't cross my mind? I'm a professor, a scholar. Theories and narratives are familiar territories, and disability as a framework wasn't far outside the boundaries I taught and studied. How could I *not* know? Eventually, naming disability added a complex, generative layer that at once deepened and illuminated my understanding of my son's embodied reality—why did it take me so long?

In this book, I've written about an interval of my life marked by constant change—an interval bookended by the beginning of silence and seizures and the end of silence and seizures.

"Beginning" started when the plan that held me together began to disintegrate. The afternoon I saw Holden's first seizure, I was seized by fear. I had no language for what was happening to my son or to my life, and I focused on making sense of it by chasing a diagnosis, contending with ever-changing medications, and grappling with the vigilance that seizure management demanded. In other words, I understood Holden's problem only as a medical one, and its only solutions rested in the hands of medical professionals. "Ending" defined itself when I developed tactics for living a more complex life. The in-between, marked by love and loss, felt profoundly disorienting. This book tells that story.

I'm not disabled—yet. I'm not yet impaired in a way that makes it difficult for me to navigate the world, not yet aged into dementia, not yet grappling with chronic pain or fatigue, not yet significantly shaped by psychosocial differences, not yet marginalized by an accident that affects my mobility. I'm not yet disabled, but this story captures how I survived the blur of my changing life, touched by my son's disability. And I'm still unlearning and relearning so I can help Holden flourish in an ableist world.[4]

Chapter One

INTERRUPTED: a process stopped

CLOSING MY OFFICE DOOR ERASED THE CHATTER OF UNDER-graduates who clustered in the hall waiting to conference with one of my colleagues. On most days, I could tune out noise: the students in the hall, my toddler playing cars in the living room, my husband's video games. But that semester, my fifth at South Dakota State University, I was teaching *Introduction to Creative Writing*, and my new version of the course foregrounded research. Excitement buzzed in my belly; I shifted in my office chair, crossing and uncrossing my legs. On the open planning document before me: *Date: / Topic: / Objectives: / Activities:*—categories meant to narrow my brainstorm.

For almost fourteen years, I'd taught writing and literature in a range of classrooms: public, private, charter, and foreign; middle schools, high schools, a community college, and three universities. Regardless of context, beginning writers almost always defined poetry as self-expression with rhymes. But poetry is more than words put in relationship because they share similar sounds. Sound must scaffold meaning and dance with the silence of white space.

How do I get beginning writers to experiment with writing from research rather than writing from emotion? I wondered. Asking them to use archival artifacts and databases to make meaning from personal experience could create some cognitive dissonance. Confronting a new teaching challenge reminded me that I, too, was still learning.

The lights in my office hummed. I turned to the four poetry bookshelves, my fingertips skimming the spines for examples to show in class—perhaps Margaret Atwood's *The Journals of Susanna Moodie* or Lee Ann Roripaugh's *Year of the Snake*. I imagined opening the next day's class with a poem on the screen. "Where do you see evidence of the poet's research?" I'd ask.[1] At first, no one would raise a hand. They'd stare at me and blink, as if unsure of their own words. A tall, blonde freshman would cock her head and smile. A bright-eyed sophomore with glasses would stare at the cellphone at the edge of his desk, hand twitching. Then someone would muster the courage to sweep away the silence with an answer.

* * *

My cellphone interrupted those thoughts. It was my son's childcare provider.

"Can you come pick up Holden right now? He's sick." I imagined my preschooler feverish, face flushed, and curled up on her lap. I sighed. *Only October*, I thought. *An early flu?*

"Does he have a fever?"

"No. But he woke up from naptime with wet jeans." Her voice shook—a new urgency from this mother of three and caretaker of ten. "And he threw up, too. On his blanket."

I pictured Holden upset by this. He always rolled his blanket up, chubby fingers against blue plush, with endearing precision.

I locked my door and headed out of the building. Outside, it was a cool day in eastern South Dakota, overcast but not threatening snow.

"And there's something else." She paused, perhaps struggling to find the words. "He won't talk. He just won't say anything."

"Really? He was chattering away this morning," I replied. Abuse, bullying, trauma—possible reasons for a child's refusing to talk—crossed my mind. Could someone be hurting him without my noticing? I drew in a sharp breath. *Slow down,* I told myself, logic intervening. Had there been evidence of abuse? No. I exhaled.

En route to pick him up, I drove past my happy places—Hillcrest Park and the Brookings city pool—and for a moment they scattered my worry. They reminded me of Lions Park in Urbandale, Iowa, where I grew up. Although Brookings—a university town of 24,000 with school in session—was more rural than the suburb of Des Moines, my life here unfolded within twenty square miles, much as it had in Urbandale.

I grew up walking to Lions Park, the Urbandale Public Library, the Hy-Vee grocery store, and St. Pius X for church on Sundays and school the rest of the week. My older sister, Theresa, and I could even walk to Merle Hay Mall in six minutes if we squeezed under a gap in a brick wall that partitioned the neighbourhood from the parking lot.

When I received a job offer from SDSU in 2007 and moved my family of three to Brookings, its similarities to Urbandale appealed to me. Its schools and parks, its trees and landscapes, even its midwestern pace and friendly atmosphere felt familiar. When I pictured raising Holden there, I hoped I could give him a similar sense of stability—just as my own childhood in Urbandale had felt.

By the time I was born in 1973, my parents and Theresa had lived there for several years, and our neighbours formed a second family. My brother, T.J., was born in 1979, and my family lived in that same house on Sixty-Sixth Street until I started my junior year of university. My dad, a quality-assurance supervisor, retired from the same company after forty years of service, and my mom elected to work outside the home only after she sent T.J. to school. I imagined our lives unfolding with that kind of stability. And for two years—until that phone call—it had.

* * *

Holden was waiting with his childcare provider when I pulled up. He grabbed my leg and hugged me as I opened her front door. I knelt down. His brown eyes were dull, and the circles under them—an inherited trait from his dad—were more pronounced than usual. I kissed his cheek. It was cool, no hint of fever.

"How are you feeling?"

He blinked but didn't speak.

I picked up the plastic bag with Holden's soiled clothes and blanket. "I'll let you know how he's feeling later," I said. "Thanks."

Holden held my hand, and we walked down the driveway. "What did you eat for lunch?" I expected, *Quesadillas!* or *A bagel!* or *Peanut butter sandwich!* He didn't respond, so I chose an alternate angle. "Did you read any dinosaur books with your friends?"

Nothing.

The day before, he'd described colouring a pumpkin, and we'd discussed possible Halloween costumes: dinosaur? superhero? ghost? He'd listed a dozen possibilities. That day I tossed out questions the whole way home: "Do you want an apple or yogurt for a snack?" "Can you sing your ABCs?" Each time silence met my questions, my stomach tightened. *He's usually so chatty*, I thought. *Why won't he speak?*

* * *

Our house sat in the pocket of a cul-de-sac. When Abel and I moved to Brookings, we bought the only house for sale that we could afford, and I loved it, even though it was a bit too far from my job at SDSU and Abel's job as a bilingual customer service representative at a credit card company. First real jobs. First home. First child. Brookings anchored us to domestic life. Soon the leaves would finish falling, and the wind would whip a neighbourhood's share into our yard. Even though we had pine trees in the front, every weekend we filled bags with leaves. Holden liked to tumble in the piles and crumble the crispest specimens in his hands.

Once inside, Holden changed into soft pants—his word for sweatpants. He was compliant, tired, silent; I was worried, driven, garrulous. I talked about anything that popped into my mind, hoping to compel a response. When nothing did, I slipped *Curious George* into the DVD player and we cuddled on the couch. The living room glowed as it did for only a few hours that time of year, sunlight slanting through the pines.

Every few minutes, when George's antics created havoc in his cartoon world, I touched Holden's forehead to check for fever.

Midway through an episode, just as George sneaked into the penguin exhibit at the zoo, Holden said, "I'm thirsty. Can I have some apple juice, please?" He looked at me and smiled.

"Coming right up!" I jumped off the couch and headed to the kitchen. "How are you feeling?"

"Great. How are you?"

"Better now that you're talking." I looked at him to see his reaction, but he was talking to Curious George: "No, George! Don't open that door. Penguins will come out!"

Words had resumed.

* * *

A few hours later, Abel walked through the door from the attached garage and waved at me as I stood over the stove.

"Hi. Be right back," he said, disappearing downstairs. Sometimes he decompressed a bit by checking his email from his computer in the basement—a catch-all level of the house: storage room, guest room, bathroom, treadmill, computer desk. The decor needed serious updating, something we'd postponed until we could afford it.

Abel resurfaced in the kitchen a few minutes later.

"How was your day?" he asked me, scooping up Holden from his circle of toys at the same time.

"Daddy!" Holden hugged him.

"It was quite an odd day, actually." I told him the story as I placed a chunk of salmon on each plate alongside broccoli and roasted sweet potatoes. I looked up to see Abel studying Holden.

"Did you get sick today at daycare?" For both of us, our default explanation was infection.

Holden nodded slowly, as if he had to think hard to summon the day.

"We played outside," he replied. "And Mommy and I watched *Curious George*!"

"That's good," Abel said.

"It was so strange." I sat down at the counter—the same place I ate, wrote poetry, coordinated schedules, and planned meals. "He just wouldn't talk."

Abel sat next to Holden. With the two of them side by side, it was easy to see the dominance of the Nuñez genes in Holden: eyes the colour of the richest chocolate bar, long eyelashes that curled at the ends, olive-toned skin. Holden had his paternal uncle's hair colour and texture, brown and wavy. Or perhaps it was a mixture of Abel's coarse black hair and my fine dishwater blonde; I didn't know much about how genes mixed.

Abel gazed at Holden for a few moments, his face soft.

"There wasn't anything else out of the ordinary?" he asked.

"No. Nothing," I replied. "That's why it's so weird. I can't think of anything that would cause him not to speak." I stammered a bit. I didn't want to inflate every concern—the worries ballooning until stress caused more damage than the concern itself. I wrestled with myself over worry.

"He doesn't seem sick now." Abel sat down on the other side of Holden, and we formed our usual triangle of talk.

Holden stabbed a broccoli floret and stuffed it into his mouth. "Broccoli. Yum!"

"Maybe the silence was just a weird fluke," I said to Abel.

"I think it was. We can just be aware, now, if we see something like it again," he replied.

* * *

I'd fallen in love with Abel at a martial arts dojo in Tempe, Arizona. He'd broken his glasses during a karate class and was MacGyvering a solution in the lobby when I arrived for a kickboxing class. We established mutual interests immediately: martial arts, which I'd begun to practise when I lived in Türkiye and which he'd been studying since high school in New Jersey; current academic pursuits at Arizona State University—mine a master's degree path in English and his a bachelor's in anthropology; and cultural appreciation in the form of good food, museums, language study, and travel.

Abel's athletic physique, gorgeous eyes, and blend of grace and strength when he practised his art attracted me, but his personality sealed it. He was unlike anyone I'd ever met: affectionate, open-minded, clever, curious, and classy. The stories of his childhood in New York City and the Dominican Republic—as the oldest of four siblings, and of his family's success as owners of three Caribbean restaurants—intrigued me. I couldn't imagine living in a huge city or on a Caribbean island; I couldn't imagine having siblings so close to me in age and dozens of cousins to grow up with. Our childhoods couldn't have been more radically different—suburban versus urban; place-stable versus transient; Midwest white versus East Coast Hispanic; Catholic school versus public school—but those differences only made us seem to fit even better.

I'm not sure how long we dated before we talked about getting married. For me, it was simply part of my life's plan—"The Plan." When I fell in love with Abel, The Plan felt intuitive, just what would happen next in the story. Growing up, I played teacher to my brother, my grandpa, and my friends; becoming an actual teacher just happened next. Reading voraciously as a child became writing books. Teaching and writing felt natural and inevitable—just what happened next—the same way I felt about wanting to marry Abel and have children.

As for Abel's plans, he didn't really have any that he shared with me. When his college adviser made him choose a major, he chose anthropology because it was the first one on the list that he liked. When I asked him what he wanted to do after graduation, and where he wanted to live, he said, "My home is with you."

* * *

When Abel suggested that we try to be more aware after Holden's silent afternoon, I agreed. Even if I hadn't been paying attention to how The Plan had manifested in my life, I'd spent years paying attention to details. They helped me manage the shadow side of my otherwise stable childhood—to sidestep the drinking habits of my father. I learned to pay attention to his face—did he seem distracted? frustrated? annoyed?—and to listen for the clink of ice cubes and the slosh of bourbon against the glass. Paying attention gave me an excuse to disappear deeper into my eight-hundred-page *World's Best Fairy Tales.* I read every book in my house (not many), including the "A" encyclopedia a salesman left for us to peruse, and my mother's high school Spanish textbook, *El Camino Real.* I paid attention in school, my curiosity and reading habits garnering good grades and welcome attention from teachers. I paid attention in church and religion classes, especially to the fascinating biographies of saints. I paid attention to my brother T.J., for whom I made worksheets and reading games. I paid attention to Theresa, whose charisma enchanted me and all who knew her; when I got older, I, too, would apply blue eye shadow, wear fashionable jeans our mother hadn't sewn, and date thick-muscled boys with winning smiles. I, too, would help people, even if it wasn't as a nurse's aide. After she started college, I even paid attention to the way Theresa made our mother cry when she came home late, or drunk, or not at all.

A life of paying attention meant I knew how to be aware. Sometimes I could sense oh-so-subtle tension, the way the body apprehends the wind's change in direction and the brain registers it as a storm brewing. Sometimes my mind would catch a paradox or chew on a juxtaposition until I put it into words—the beginning of a poem. Then I would take inventories of examples and associations, building lines with imagery.[2] Paying attention was something I could do.

And yet. Just as storm clouds gather and dissipate before producing a drop of rain, I forgot about Holden's silent afternoon until fear unsettled my memory.

* * *

"Yeeee-haw! Courtesy of your friendly neighbourhood Spider-Man!" a recorded voice sprang up from the living room.

"Do you like your new toy, Holden?" I was scrubbing frosting from his birthday cake off a plate, my hands immersed in suds. Holden didn't reply. "That's such a great action figure!" Glancing over my shoulder, I saw him lying on the couch, Spider-Man resting on the floor beneath his open hand. A chaos of paper and ribbons littered the floor; *Pin the*

Spider-Man on the Web, Silly String games, and "run around until you fall down" had exhausted kids and parents alike. Abel followed my gaze.

"I'll take him to his bedroom," Abel said. "He's probably exhausted from the party."

But he returned from Holden's room, perplexed. "It's strange. He's sleeping with his eyes open." Abel's voice sounded strained.

I dried my hands on my jeans. As I walked into his room, I recalled stories my mother told of Theresa sleeping with her eyes open when she was a toddler. I imagined Holden's heavy-lidded eyes closing slowly yet revealing irises below the eyelashes, like my childhood baby doll.

But Holden was staring straight ahead. His face was tense, and his body was rigid. I rubbed his shoulder. "Holden, sweetie. Hey." No response. "Holden! Let's go play with your new toys."

No sigh.

No rollover.

No eye movement.

I looked at his chest. Did I see breathing, or did I just imagine it? I gasped, then picked him up under his armpits and gently shook him. Nothing changed.

"I can't tell if he's breathing!" I yelled, carrying him out to the living room. "I'm calling 911."

I handed Holden to Abel and tapped in the number. As I answered the standard questions from the operator—What's your name? What's your son's name?—panic rose. I didn't know what was coming next—yet I did.

Something unspeakable.

Something out of my control.

Something I must endure.

My stomach released, and nausea pitched me forward as the memory surfaced. The morning of November 13, 1984: sirens pulled me out of sleep; my father stood outside our front door in his flannel robe, whispering, "They can't find her pulse."

My mother had found her oldest daughter asphyxiated, the car's engine still running.

Theresa was dead.

* * *

As I hung up the phone and waited for the paramedics, I felt the full weight of that memory—and the grief that followed. All I could do was stand next to Abel while he steadied our son on the kitchen counter. Then, just as I heard sirens, Holden's abdomen moved. He groaned. A wet stain formed on his jeans as he rolled over and vomited. My body tensed up again. He wasn't dead—but was he dying?

The paramedics swept into the room.

"Put him on the floor," one said. I shoved gift boxes and wrapping paper to the side. One took Holden's pulse while the other shined a flashlight into his eyes.

"What's your name, buddy?" the one with the flashlight asked. No response. "How old are you?" Still nothing.

I knelt next to Holden and held his hand. He seemed conscious. His heart was beating. *They thought Theresa's heart was beating at first, too*, I heard a voice inside me say. I shook my head, as if doing so could make it untrue.

"Your son had a seizure." The paramedic stood up and stretched a bit. "He's fine now, but a doctor should examine him."

The edges of my vision blurred. He hadn't twitched or convulsed, so how could it have been a seizure? I knew seizures only from a story Theresa had told me. During her part-time job in her senior year of high school, she'd worked at a daycare, and a child had seized in her arms—his eyes rolling back. She held him while another teacher put a spoon in his mouth so he wouldn't swallow his tongue. When it ended, he was fine. Theresa told the story dramatically, but I'd seen the fear behind her eyes.

The paramedics took Holden to the hospital for observation. Abel and I followed in our car. The paramedics who came to my childhood home had allowed my mother to go with them, but they'd left my father alone. With Holden safe in the hands of professionals, I was grateful Abel and I weren't separated. During the five-minute drive, we stumbled over our words, recounting bits of what we'd just seen. Only an hour earlier, the concept of a seizure had been hazy—like a word I could use in a sentence but not define. They happened to other people, like a grey sky far off on the horizon meant someone else would need to take shelter from a storm or escape a burning building.

At the forty-nine-bed hospital, a physician assistant examined Holden, who was sleepy, silent, and be-stickered with superheroes on his shirt. Under the bright lights, IV fluids eased into his body. The P.A. ordered a CT scan to rule out an obvious cause for the seizure, such as a tumour. When the scan didn't reveal anything concerning, the P.A. speculated that an influx of sugar from the birthday cake and ice cream had triggered it. Holden's ears looked a little red, too. He prescribed antibiotics for an ear infection, even though Holden wasn't running a fever. We left with an appointment card for our primary care physician, a prescription, and a pamphlet.

On the way home, I thought about the range of extremes presented as explanations for the seizure. It was either something simple and easily avoided again—too much sugar—or something life-threatening, like a tumour. The seizure first aid pamphlet listed common causes—lack of sleep, sugar influx, fever—but none felt right. I considered Holden's sleeping schedule; he seemed to get a full night's rest. I recalled putting the cake and ice cream on his plate at his party, but it had been a modest slice. *Something's missing*, I thought. *I'm missing something.*

Then I remembered. "We don't diagnose epilepsy unless he has more than one seizure," the P.A. had said. *More than one. More than one.*

That day in October—just three months ago—when I picked him up from childcare. Vomit. Urination. Not speaking for hours.

"Oh my God, Abel. Wow. Oh my God. This probably wasn't his first seizure." I could barely speak fast enough. "Remember that afternoon at daycare? In October? This was his second." As I compared the events—the similarities obvious—a flicker of anger rose. How could I have forgotten until now? Would remembering have made a difference at the ER? Abel reassured me that it wouldn't have, so I calmed down, promising myself to explain it all to his family doctor when we saw her later that week.

* * *

The fear of seizures and the fear of unknown futures commingled that night. I didn't know enough about epilepsy to defuse the first.[3] I didn't know what various types of seizures could look like; I didn't know a child could have one during naptime at the babysitter's house or after his birthday party; I didn't know a seizure could make him vomit and urinate; I didn't know that my post-seizure son might not have the energy to speak for hours; I didn't know that he couldn't describe tumbling off the precipice of consciousness. If I didn't have words for it, how could he? And what I did know about seizures was myth—spoons and swallowing tongues. What other things did I think I knew but got wrong?

I did know something about how futures could shift from watching my mother grieve. She watched to see whether her child was breathing; she called emergency services; she waited with doctors for answers. The coroner ruled Theresa's death accidental because her blood-alcohol level was so high that she couldn't have chosen suicide with a clear mind, even if that had been her intention. My family and I imagined that she fell asleep listening to her favourite song on the radio after coming home from the bar. Our garage had only one door, so she would have had to shut it manually and slip back into her car to do that. And why would she do that? But there wasn't a note or previous attempts. No one knew if she'd been depressed.

After the shock and numbness wore off, I vowed not to let Theresa's death be *in vain*. I'd live enough for both of us. I'd transform into a beautiful, charismatic extrovert who loved to help people, and I'd learn to avoid her mistakes. I wouldn't drink; I wouldn't party. The summer before eighth grade, I wrote up lists for self-improvement. *Seventeen* magazine instructed me on hairstyles and lipstick selection. I generously applied Sun-In. I memorized ways to meet boys and make more friends. Drawing myself out of the painful shell of my life meant shaving off a storyline from Theresa's and merging it with mine.

For years, plans seemed to work. And yet now illness threatened my stable life. Fears mingled, and a sense of disruption lingered. My only insight? Two seizures make a pattern—and patterns always mean something.

Chapter Two

INTERCEPT: to seize en route

A SEIZURE OCCURS WHEN COMPLEX CHEMICAL CHANGES OCCURring in nerve cells cause a sudden surge of electrical activity—a brainstorm. One neurologist, Douglas R. Labar, explained to *New York Times* reporter Denise Grady how seizures occur. Whereas most of the time groups of neurons act independently, during a seizure, large groups of neurons fire together: they sync up and act in an "abnormally repetitive, fast way." He also compared a seizure to "fans doing the wave in a stadium."[1] In this 2004 article, "Doctors Put Hope in Thin Wires to Ease the Clutches of Epilepsy," Grady presents interviews from neurologists across the United States regarding the use of stimulators designed to decrease seizure activity in patients with intractable epilepsy—when seizures cannot be prevented by medication. The article highlights the fear surrounding seizures. Grady quotes neurologist Ivan Osorio: "Epilepsy is the most elusive and most treacherous of neurological diseases, because of its intermittency, and also the cruelest, because you never know when it is going to strike next." Dr. Osorio compares a seizure to fire "spreading through the brain."[2]

The seizure that occurred on the day we celebrated Holden's fourth birthday ignited this sense of treacherous fear, and the fear moved along the paths forged by grief. I worried that I'd lose Holden just as my parents lost Theresa. Most parents want to protect their children, but this fear felt primal and expansive. It simmered just below the surface, shaping my decisions. It lurked at the edges of my consciousness, influencing me without awareness. Even as I waited for an official diagnosis, the factors that sparked fear were waiting—ready to sync up, ready to fire together, ready to seize me.

* * *

The week following the birthday seizure, Holden's family doctor recommended a sleep–wake electroencephalogram (EEG).[3] The solemnity with which she discussed the test did nothing to assuage my fear. During the EEG, Holden stayed hooked up to the brain wave sensors (electrodes) for two hours while awake and for two hours while asleep. When the results indicated abnormal brain activity, our family doctor referred us to a pediatric neurologist in Sioux Falls—a forty-five-minute drive south from our home in Brookings.

Even though Sioux Falls was the largest city in South Dakota, the earliest appointment we could get for Holden was five weeks out, at the very end of February. Five weeks. Five weeks to conduct some basic research on epilepsy—reading intended to soothe my anxiety. Five weeks to maintain my teaching and meet a book-manuscript deadline. Five weeks to stew in worry and waiting: Would he seize again?

I took some solace in routines. Confident that Holden's daycare provider kept a close eye on him, I drilled down into work as soon as I dropped him off. After finishing up a prepping/teaching/grading cycle, I worked on proofreading *Keeping Them Alive*, a book that braids poems inspired by Holden's birth and Theresa's death. The poems about Theresa start with the day of her death—the rest beads on a string of grief. To counterpoint, the poems about Holden start with anticipating conception, followed by pregnancy, birth, and infancy. I'd determined the book's arrangement long before Holden's seizure, but as I read through them again, the twist of these two strands emphasized the motherhood theme. The fear of possibly losing Holden and the grief from confronting Theresa's death made it difficult to concentrate. When I came to a poem about the impact of Theresa's death on my mother, I imagined that happening to me—and I had to stop working on the manuscript.

When anxiety fuzzed my focus, I pushed poetry aside and read about epilepsy. The impression that I could learn my way into comfort held sway. Browsing the Epilepsy Foundation's website, I learned that seizures could cause abnormal physical behaviours, like chewing motions or dropping to the ground. I read that one in twenty-six people in the United States will develop epilepsy in their lifetime; more than 65 million people globally have active epilepsy. Medical professionals prefer the term "seizure disorder" because it describes the diagnosis better than "epilepsy." Genetics, head trauma, infectious diseases, brain conditions, strokes, and prenatal injuries can all cause seizures, but many people diagnosed with epilepsy have no clear indication about its cause. Medications control seizures for many, but others need surgery or significant dietary change. And for others, no medical solutions work.[4]

Not once do I remember reading the word "disability" associated with epilepsy.

I gleaned advice on seizure first aid. Friends, family—even strangers—can keep a person from hitting their head if they drop to the ground. They can remove objects nearby to keep the seizing individual from striking their head. Turning the person on their side can help if they vomit. Myths were busted up, too: under no circumstances should a person put something in the mouth of a seizing individual. They can't swallow their tongues. They shouldn't be restrained.

And yet when I fell down these research rabbit holes, I always got stuck. One click beyond "Epilepsy 101" introduced jargon: *generic drug equivalence* (they're not always equivalent?), *rare epilepsy network* (there's more than one type of epilepsy?), and *SUDEP Institute* (acronyms, acronyms, and more acronyms). The more specific the information, the more confused I became. Awash with new ideas and the emotions they elicited, I followed the same impulse that Theresa's death had sparked in me: I wrote. I ruminated with images and fragments:

Electrical activity, seizures as lightning storms, open-prairie thunderstorms.

Grey matter is a giant cluster of rainclouds.

Connecting cells snap like lightning bolts, and a horizon of bolts branches out. For a few minutes, they control behaviour—what hands do, what eyes do. Then the lightning burns itself out, leaving the air cool and spent.

When I look at Holden's hair, I imagine a labyrinth of fatty acid molecules beneath skin and skull.

Holden's brain is a sky I can't see, a sky I can't hold.

Writing poetic fragments created an associative space for me to think through images, which made abstract phenomena a bit more concrete for me. It also helped me articulate my emotions, albeit obliquely—storms of any sort felt destructive and scary. Slowing down the process as I learned new information, writing gave me a way to track concepts even if I couldn't understand everything right away. Later, I would pick up these fragments and piece them together, artifacts of my own learning.

In the short term, my reading pinned me between fearing seizures and not knowing exactly what about them I should fear. Even though website authors emphasized that most people don't die from seizures, fear reigned: *What if I can't get to him fast enough to protect his head? What if I'm not there? What if he has a seizure in his sleep?*

This research process felt like trudging through a desert, exhausted by heat but lured by mirages. I searched site after site for answers, for clarity. An occasional glimmer—a sentence that would make sense in Holden's case—often dissipated into vagueness. I collected concepts, but interpreting them derailed me. Chronic illness, for example. What did that mean, exactly? Would Holden be considered chronically ill? What criteria applied? If so, what did that mean for him? What did that mean for me? As a professor, research that resulted in headaches wasn't new, but the pressure of what was at stake—keeping Holden safe—overwhelmed me.

Abel didn't seem to share my worry, but perhaps he just didn't share his worries with me. In the evenings, after eating dinner, playing with Holden, and tucking him into bed, we would binge a favourite television series. We'd established that habit when I was in graduate school, usually saving the best ones for weekends. I looked forward to curling into his arms and surrendering my thoughts to whatever series he'd queued up. Abel was generous with affection and tenderness and touch. Sometimes he could relax my churning mind with a simple backrub or a deep embrace.

Other times, I couldn't help but process my worries out loud. On those evenings, before he pressed play on the remote, I'd share the questions I had about epilepsy. He'd listen attentively, but he didn't add much. He knew the situation was beyond "everything will be okay," yet he didn't seem to have a grip on it either. I wanted us to research together, or, since that wasn't happening, pool the inquiries we conducted separately. Abel tended to stay up a few hours later than I did every night. If he used that time for research, I hoped he'd share it. But it seemed as if the initial research he'd conducted the night of the birthday seizure satisfied him. So when I failed to get him to share his thoughts, I snuggled with him in front of the screen.

* * *

When Holden's neurology appointment finally arrived at the end of February, my expectations were high. I imagined the neurologist would explain what epilepsy meant for Holden. I imagined she would answer the questions I had and the questions that bubbled up in our rich conversation. I imagined leaving confident, with a plan to stop Holden's seizures so I could focus on my routines without fear surfacing.

Holden expressed his own excitement when he saw the blue-topped conical spires and white brick of the children's hospital in Sioux Falls.

"It looks like a castle," Holden said. "What is this place?" Inside, we peered at murals of knights and brightly painted animals before enduring the usual check-in procedures. On our way to the room, the nurse measured his weight, height, and blood pressure. The diagnostic tools I associated with check-ups or infections surprised me. And yet why did I think a visit to a neurologist should proceed any differently? I had absolutely no experience.

Abel was reading *Hop on Pop* to Holden when a woman about my age walked into the room. Bright smile. Bright eyes. Confident.

"Hello, I'm Helen, Dr. Porter's assistant. I'm a nurse practitioner." She extended her hand to shake mine, then Abel's. "You'll see Dr. Porter during your next visit in six months."

Silence hung in the air.

"So ... we're not going to meet Dr. Porter today?" I asked.

"No. But she goes over each case carefully with me."

Doubt snagged my thoughts. Epilepsy seemed so complex, and this system seemed so indirect.

Helen sat down in a chair opposite me. "Has Holden had any more seizures?"

"No," I said, shaking my head. Abel did the same.

"Okay. Good. So the pattern on Holden's EEG indicates that he has a seizure disorder," Helen said. She asked if we were familiar with the terms *grand mal* and *petit mal* to describe kinds of seizures. We both nodded yes. Then she explained that these terms were outdated. The kind she thought Holden had most often was absence seizures. I remembered them from my research: brief yet repeated moments of lost consciousness. They didn't feature convulsions.

"Typical absence seizures are less than ten seconds long and are easily controlled by medication," Helen said. "They're normally outgrown by adulthood."

"Absence seizures? Really?" I tried to recall seeing one. "I guess he does space out from time to time." Still, I hadn't noticed anything as profound as daily seizures. His childcare provider and his preschool teachers hadn't mentioned any concerns either. "But wasn't the January seizure bigger?"

"Yes," Helen nodded. "Sometimes people experience a mixed bag of seizures. That January episode was a complex partial seizure—what people used to call a grand mal seizure. The Depakote Dr. Porter's prescribing should cover both kinds."[5]

Mixed bag? I imagined a plastic grocery bag with a range of seizures inside. Skittles candies—the absence kind. Watermelon—a bigger kind. A pomegranate, four popcorn balls, three grapefruit, a handful of

Oreos—kinds she implied existed. So the EEG showed absence seizure activity, but he also had a different kind too? Did the EEG convey anything about that? I was confused, and yet I didn't know what to ask. Abel didn't seem to either. A ripple of frustration flashed through me. I felt rushed, and I didn't know how to formulate my doubt and confusion as questions.

"Give him showers, not baths. Don't let him swim alone. Have teachers watch him on the playground equipment. And steer him away from professions where heights factor in, like construction management." Helen smiled; she'd given this speech before. I tasted a sour annoyance. Was epilepsy really not a big deal? Not a chronic illness? Had the fear caused me to overreact? I couldn't think of a reason why this wasn't the right course of action, and yet I wasn't persuaded by her implications that our lives wouldn't change much beyond an increased awareness of playground safety and a capsule of Depakote sprinkles twice a day. Still, I dabbed my doubts with her comfort: this was the most treatable form of epilepsy.

Helen handed us a prescription. The main side effect of Depakote to worry about, she explained, was a liver problem, but a blood draw in a few weeks would rule that out. She also prescribed Diastat, an emergency seizure medication for the watermelon-sized seizures that lasted more than three minutes. "Most people won't need to use the Diastat, but keep it on hand, just in case. It's a suppository," she said. I nodded. "As for the Depakote, we start children at the lowest dose and will want blood drawn for that too, to see if it's reached a therapeutic level. You can have all lab work done in Brookings, and they will fax the results to us."

"Okay," I responded, dazed by this new layer of information. Side effects. Side effects one might not be able to observe visually but only know about via lab work.

"Call us if he has another seizure," Helen said. "And we can increase the Depakote dose." She closed her laptop and sat forward in her chair.

I felt stunned, so when neither Abel nor I summoned a question, we thanked her and ushered Holden through the hallways so we could go home.[6]

* * *

One of the most studied models of epilepsy is called *kindling*.[7] When I first read "kindling," conducting research in fits and starts as a mother under duress, I pictured the flames in my family's fireplace—newspaper as kindling. I can still hear the match strike as my fingers pulled it across the red strip; then, tip touched paper. Flame. Ash.

But in epilepsy, kindling is less about fire and more about movement. It refers to a pattern of movement and the effect of that pattern. In the kindling model, successive seizures move along the same brain circuitry and create a path that future seizures take. Over time, more seizures and more intense seizures happen along these routes. Neural desire lines. Lightning storms where multiple strikes happen in the same place. Kindling is also a good metaphor for the way I experienced the movement of fear and how it seized me—at first hovering, then kindled by a spark of memory or ignited by crisis.

When I began conducting research as a scholar in disability studies nearly a decade after Holden's first seizure, I found Aurora Levins Morales's *Kindling: Writings on the Body*. In this book, Morales describes how scientists repeatedly stimulate the brains of animals to cause seizures, which permanently lowers their seizure thresholds. That means seizures happen more often. Further, she explains that parts of the brain—the amygdala (integrative centre for emotions), the hippocampus (responsible for learning and memory), and the cortex (outer layer), as well as receptors for particular neurotransmitters—actually change as a result of repeated stimulation. Recurring seizures can result in the death of neurons and injury to nerve cells. These changes can also lead "to a state of cellular hyper-excitability" with "signs of increased anxiety, depression, and cognitive problems" in kindled brains.[8]

Morales's work helped me understand the possible effects of repeated seizures on a person's brain, but it also gave me a metaphor for my own emotional reality. My fear shuttled me into worry and precluded the possibility of multiple, complex, and layered answers. I wonder now whether having this awareness sooner would've interrupted my narrow thinking process. Perhaps after fear kindled, I could have named what was happening instead of freezing with confusion, unable to ask questions or articulate my concerns. I must reflect now, well over a decade after Holden's epilepsy diagnosis, because I want to understand how my own patterns hindered my ability to be a better advocate for my child, and how ableist systems reinforced my status quo. No medical professional directed me to resources that could help me think about Holden's epilepsy diagnosis in other ways or offered resources that could better prepare me for possibilities.

If I'd known about Morales's work when I'd walked into Dr. Porter's office—or even writers like Morales who approached chronic health conditions from a disability perspective— perhaps I would have considered more nuanced ways of understanding epilepsy. Perhaps I would have been invited not to expect a neurologist to have all the answers, or been asked to question my faith in medicine to have the clear and right answers. Perhaps I would have been better prepared to see the signs of increased anxiety, depression, and cognitive problems that would emerge later in my son.

In *Kindling*, Morales not only illustrates how she grapples with the physical and mental effects of seizures, she also explores disability, pain, and healing in the context of her body, our collective body, and the body of the planet. These connected sites need attention and care, and she argues that considering individuals affected by environmental change will help us understand how to move forward. "My body and your bodies make a map we can follow," she writes.[9] Morales also argues that various therapies—art, writing, collaboration—contribute to wellness, and models how to question medical professionals even as she stays open to what they can provide.

Instead, rigid in my thinking, I sought a literal map on how to move forward with the epilepsy diagnosis. And I'd wanted the neurologist to provide it. Why did I give Helen—Dr. Porter's stand-in—this responsibility? Because she was a product of rigorous training, and a person for whom (I assumed) seizure disorders lacked mystery. I thought she'd be the one to tell me what I needed to know. Perhaps she thought it wasn't her job to help me understand; a prescription plus orders for lab work equalled problem solved. Perhaps she just assumed I understood or would seek out additional understanding on my own.

* * *

During the month of March, I wanted to believe that with this prescription, our usual routines could resume. And yet, I also looked for the kind of seizures Helen said Holden experienced. I searched for them on his face when he played, ate, and watched TV. When he sat on a kitchen stool and began to build a tower of LEGO bricks, I watched: yellow on green, green on red, blue on yellow. Up, up, up—he'd stack bricks one at a time. Then, he might pause, LEGO brick midair.

"Holden!" My chest would fill with worry.

"Yes?" He'd add the brick. Was that a quick spell or a daydream? Every time I thought I saw an absence seizure, he always responded. Perhaps he was just thinking.

And then I'd wonder. The difference between an absence seizure and a daydream seemed semantic if the episode was singular, not multiple in quick succession. If they were seizures, they'd stack like the LEGO tower, creating a reality-skipping effect—as if his mind were a broken movie projector. I blinked my eyes to mimic that effect, but I couldn't eclipse the sensation of continued consciousness. The lost consciousness of a seizure could mean a fall from a swing, a trip down the stairs, or a slip underwater in the bathtub. It could mean Holden's inability to avoid a speeding car. These seizures mattered, and I needed to figure them out.

The more I read about seizures, the more I pictured them as a blend of tornado and lightning storm—perhaps because massive storms felt extreme, an analogue to what was happening in Holden's brain, or perhaps because they rendered humans helpless for a while—that, too, like Holden. During my childhood, when tornado sirens went off and the sky turned yellow-green, it meant a tornado could drop at any second. I wrote in my notebook, *A fever precedes a seizure like yellow-green skies precede tornadoes.* Through association, I sought comprehension.

I wrote under those yellow-green skies and watched Holden spill out his LEGO bin. I waited for the roof to fly off the house, for the windows to shatter, for the linden to be lifted from the ground. Instead, he'd return to his LEGO. As the number of days Holden took the Depakote increased, I hoped that I wasn't seeing seizures because the medicine had erased them. A friend bolstered my faith in that notion when she told me her son had used Depakote successfully and without side effects. Nine years older than Holden, he'd only ever had two seizures and outgrew the medication. I felt a tug of reassurance that it was working just as Helen said it would. Certainly, the seizures were behind us.

* * *

I was wrong. In April, just five weeks after the visit with Helen, Holden seized again. We were driving home after spending Easter weekend with my parents in Iowa. That morning, he'd run out of his bedroom with a basket in hand, then hunted for eggs in the backyard, finding them in low tree branches or behind flowerpots. He giggled as he hustled from spot to spot. "Another egg! Look! A blue one!" Afterward, he walked up with a full basket and complained that his stomach hurt. His head felt warm. I moved to worry mode. If he was getting sick, I preferred to be at home and close to his doctor. We grabbed our stuff, hopped into the car, and headed north.

Three hours into the trip, between bits of song and conversation, Holden stopped chatting. When he didn't speak for a minute, I turned around. His eyes were locked sideways. I said his name and snapped my fingers in front of his face. He didn't respond.

"He's having a seizure. Pull over!" Click. Seat belt off. My research lacked scenarios for *Seizure Response on the Interstate*. The car slowed down but didn't stop. My muscles tensed. Adrenaline ramped up my heart rate.

"Is there an exit ramp close? A town? Something safe?" Abel asked. He was right. The shoulder was a dangerous place to stop, but the next exit could've been fifteen miles away.

"I don't know," I said. "We could keep driving and see if he stops, or we could pull over to take him out of the car." Which was safest? If he vomited sitting up, it might not drain from his mouth. "I think you should pull over now."

Abel moved to the shoulder and pressed the hazard button. I jumped out, unbuckled Holden, and carried him into the ditch. Crouching in the snow, I eased him onto his left side as the first aid videos described.

My body swayed. The sky was bright blue, but the wind cut through my spring jacket. Broken cornstalks poked through snow, thinned drifts revealing rich soil. Behind us, eighteen-wheelers roared past at ninety miles an hour. Abel hovered near the car.

"How long will this last?" I looked into Holden's vacant eyes. Then I realized I hadn't been timing the length of the seizure. And I hadn't brought the emergency medication either.

Since our appointment in Sioux Falls, I'd stuffed the zip-close box—double the width of an eyeglass case and three inches longer—into my purse before every outing with Holden. I'd grown accustomed to seeing *Diastat AcuDial* (diazepam rectal gel) embossed on the black case as I shoved it out of the way to make room for a book or juice box or snack bag. Inside was a large tube of medication with a plastic three-inch taper at one end and a plunger at the other. The amount was "dialled up" for proper administration. But I hadn't remembered to put it back in my purse before the trip. This life-saving medicine was on top of our refrigerator.

After his diagnosis, I often mentally rehearsed what would happen if Holden seized in public: at the grocery store, Holden would collapse in front of a display of cauliflower. I'd keep my composure and time the seizure, putting my body between him and the strangers who would undoubtedly gather. If the seizure lasted too long, I'd pull off his jeans and give him the medicine. But sometimes I stumbled: Would I remember to apply the packet of lubricating jelly before inserting the suppository? It seemed too private for a public place. Embarrassed by even imagining this scenario, I also felt ashamed for feeling embarrassed, so I psyched myself up. *You're a mom. Moms must muster strength,* I thought. When Theresa died, my mom had planned her funeral, picked out a headstone, and confronted everyone's grief; my challenge was so small in comparison.

I hated myself for forgetting the Diastat, and I hated myself for assuming the Depakote had been working. I rocked Holden a bit faster. "You'll be fine in a minute," I whispered. "You'll be fine." Did falling into a seizure frighten Holden? Did he think he was dying? Did it hurt? I panicked at the possibilities, and I wanted to absorb Holden's fear.

I didn't have a plan for what would happen if three minutes passed and he was still seizing. I wondered if Abel did. I wondered where Abel was.

At my twentieth "You'll be fine," Holden squeezed my elbow. The seizure was over. I hugged him and stood up. When Abel saw me staggering through the ditch, he hustled to help.

I sensed no judgment from Abel when I admitted I'd forgotten the emergency medication. The only anger present was my own. For the rest of the drive, I sorted through relief that Holden had recovered and anger at my own mistake. I'd dropped my vigilance. I'd been tested, and I blew it.

* * *

Another seizure would happen a few weeks later, in mid-May—longer and more dramatic than the one on the highway. I referred to it as epic. Abel heard an odd noise on the baby monitor we'd put back in Holden's room. He checked on Holden and found him seizing in bed. When I arrived, I put my hand on his forehead; he was burning up. Since we didn't know when the seizure had started, I ran to get the Diastat. Abel carried Holden from his bed to the bathroom and placed him in the empty bathtub. It seemed logical—Holden might urinate or vomit. We both stood there, my arm poised to hand Abel the Diastat or administer it to Holden myself.

I felt prepared to act until I saw Holden continue to convulse.

No amount of first aid knowledge could tamp down the fear that he could die. The energy swirling in my chest dropped into my stomach. I sank to my knees.

No amount of readiness could facilitate my body's movements. In this tornado's eye, I was caught. The chaos of the seizure felt like a churning wall of cloud, my own body—still in the centre—illuminated by a bluish light. Abel soothed Holden as he supported him in the tub, the words twisting from his mouth and spinning away. Somewhere overhead, bursts of lightning urged me to move. In those few seconds, fear shocked me into silence.

Then Holden's abdomen clenched. Vomit squirted out his nose. Panic resolved my suspension and flooded my limbs. I felt the familiar tingling—the electricity of potential. My senses sharpened, and I leaned forward to examine him. His facial muscles were tensed, his jaw locked shut. *What's happening?* I thought. The seizure wasn't stopping.

"Time for the Diastat," I said. Abel took the syringe from my hand. We worked in sync. "I'll call 911." I turned out of the room.

Abel administered the Diastat while I was on the phone. The seizure subsided less than a minute later. Holden started to breathe normally just as the paramedics arrived.

"You put him in the tub? That's not a good idea," one of them scolded us as she lifted him out. She explained that Holden could've smacked his head against the side and knocked himself out, complicating the seizure. His position in the tub also prevented us from securing his arms and legs and keeping him on his side. I hung my head, embarrassed. It seemed so obvious. At least she'd said something—otherwise how would we know? *You've got to chase the knowledge,* I thought. Guilt turned my stomach.

Holden's pale complexion, high fever, and lethargy alarmed the paramedics. They checked his vital signs and decided to take him to the hospital. "Just to be safe," one said, "and monitor his reaction to the Diastat." Some people had an allergic reaction, he explained. Since this was Holden's first use of it, observing him for a few hours would be prudent. I made a mental note: double-check the side effects of the emergency medication.

Holden's ER visit was much like his first. He lay in the hospital bed, exhausted, IV hooked up. He didn't say a word—not to get a sticker, not to get chocolate pudding, not to make the nurses laugh. He slept until Tylenol brought his 103.5°F mystery fever down. But he had handled the Diastat well. And when we were finally discharged at 3:00 a.m., Holden took one step out of the hospital and yelled, "Yahoo!" Again, his words resumed. I exhaled some stress, and I laughed out loud.

* * *

Just five months—from January to May—presented me with a series of my son's seizures to pin on a blank page. I attempted to connect the dots, but moments of terror gripped me at random times. The image of Holden seizing in the tub flashed in front of me when I was in the shower, prepping a meal, or on a walk. After the epic seizure in May, fear seized me more often and with greater intensity. When the panic passed, I sorted through what I could do to check on Holden. Bound out of the shower? Call his childcare provider? Ask Abel how Holden was doing in the next room? I wrestled with myself over what to do, how to do it, and then even whether I should do it. *You can't call the daycare so much in the day; there are kids to take care of,* I thought. *Abel knows what he's doing; he's his dad.*

And looking to research no longer felt comforting. What caused the abnormal neuron activity mystified me. Gaining a deeper understanding meant learning a new language: glial cells, synapses, dendrites, axons, frontal lobe, cerebral cortex. A seizure threshold meant the balance between excitatory and inhibitory forces in the brain that affect how susceptible a person is to seizures, but how could I control all the factors—fever, high stress, sleep deprivation, flashing or flickering lights, and exhaustion—that could affect Holden? What were Holden's triggers, exactly? What stressed him out, and how would I know when it was too much?[10]

I saw myself when I read Morales's chapter "Coming Out Sick": "In that world of impending shipwrecks, avoiding the tips of icebergs was enough to handle."[11] Morales needed to take care of herself, which included intense, all-night sessions conducting research into her symptoms as well as taking care of her aging father. She describes herself as struggling to balance his needs with her own. I hadn't quite come to that exhausted sense of drowning, but I'd begun to feel the cold wind blowing. Anxiety and fear reinforced that frozen feeling, and I'd begun to feel slow to act.

I wish I'd known that grappling with Holden's seizure disorder—keeping him safe—was part of a larger challenge for me: confronting the dissolution of The Plan. The kindling of fear reinforced my rigidity.

The routines that once provided structure and security didn't consistently do that anymore, but I couldn't yet let go of them.

So I took inventory of what I did know. I knew enough to be terrified of seizures—terrified of their randomness, their range of presentation, their stealth. I knew that medicine could mitigate them—sometimes. I knew that fevers and other phenomena could lower seizure thresholds. I knew when and how to give the Diastat. But for each shred of knowledge I asserted, I countered it. I criticized myself for not moving faster and more decisively with the Diastat; I criticized myself for not understanding the disease mechanism better, for not absorbing the medical research more quickly; I criticized myself for not anticipating all the possible dangers.

Spinning in these cycles of thinking, I doubted my ability to be a good mom. I doubted my ability to keep Holden safe. I doubted my ability to keep Holden alive.

Chapter Three

INTERTWINED: twisted together

THE DAY OF HOLDEN'S MID-JANUARY SEIZURE, EXHAUSTED after prepping for his fourth birthday party, I'd supposed I was pregnant. The drama of the seizure distracted me that week, but then a pregnancy test at the end of the month confirmed it. Even while I worried, mini-movies of Holden and his future sibling popped up: Holden's hand on my round belly as I read his favourite book; Holden cradling a swaddled bundle, bits of brown hair framing the baby's face; big brother shaking a rattle at the little one while we snuggled on the couch; Holden making silly faces for his sibling while riding in the car; Holden scooting his high chair next to the baby's so he could help spoon sweet potato.

I wanted a second child because I loved being a mom. I marvelled at watching Holden learn, from finding his toes to knowing which sounds animals make. And he was a fun kid. Holden loved to play from the moment he woke up. After he turned one, he invented a new eating game where he put a piece of food between us, then placed it in his own mouth with a big laugh. His favourite toys were those he invented from plastic bottles, cups filled with lentils, and the KitchenAid mixer bowl (it becomes a bell when struck with a wooden spoon). I cherished the quiet moments too. When we cuddled up to read books, he gripped his blanket with one hand and Purple Bunny, a soft rattle-like toy, with the other. When he "read along" with me, pointing to the words on the page, I felt a surge of joy. If having one child could be this heart-expanding, why not two?

Holden had just turned two when Abel and I started to discuss adding another child. Abel said he was *almost* ready. The first time around, our conversations about trying to conceive centred not on whether we wanted a child (we did) but on the timing. Abel worried about money; he wanted me to finish school and find a job first. But I was worried about how long it might take to have a baby. I was twenty-nine when I started the doctoral program. With my coursework done, I still needed to finish my comprehensive exams. When I mentioned plans to conceive with my doctor, she must've picked up on my wish to perfectly time the pregnancy because I recall her telling me that the average woman takes two years to conceive. My mother had trouble conceiving after Theresa was born, which gave me another reason to start trying. We conceived Holden the second month into the endeavour.

When we discussed adding another child, we considered the financial implications of additional daycare and the logistics of scheduling another person's needs. We assumed we already knew what those needs would be: diaper changes, feedings every two hours, trips to the doctor for ear infections. We circled around those anticipated changes for several weeks before Abel resolved his indecision.

I was sitting on the living room floor reading to Holden when I looked up to see Abel smiling. "What are you thinking?" I asked.

"About having another baby," he replied.

I imagined another quick conception. Instead, it took me seven months to get pregnant, and then I quickly miscarried. I didn't even have the opportunity to use the early pregnancy test I'd bought. Bleeding and cramping after I'd thought my period had ended sent me to urgent care. A blood test there confirmed pregnancy, but miscarriage seemed likely, and another round of blood work two days later revealed that pregnancy hormone levels had dropped. I was disappointed but not devastated. I knew a few women who'd had a miscarriage, so this seemed like a possible part of the process. At age thirty-four, I believed the dominant narratives about age and motherhood: the longer one waits, the harder it becomes to conceive. And yet, I felt young, and I felt fertile.

A second miscarriage happened the same summer that Abel, Holden, and I visited Krakow, Prague, and Munich—a full year after the first. For one week in late July, I knew I was pregnant; then one morning I started bleeding. My hand shook as I held the phone and described what was happening to my doctor. She told me to come to the clinic, and there she confirmed the miscarriage. When I asked her why it had happened *again*, she said it wasn't my fault. Still, I obsessed over all the ways I'd behaved—abstaining from alcohol and soft cheeses, avoiding the cat's litter box—as I searched for any change I could make for the next time to feel absolutely certain that I hadn't done anything wrong.[1]

* * *

Despite the stress of Holden's fourth-birthday-party seizure, waiting for that first EEG, and absorbing the diagnosis from Helen, when I found out I was pregnant again, I felt optimistic. Every day, I took a deep breath and passed my hand over my belly with a quick prayer: *Grow healthy, grow strong, grow whole.* Eight weeks in, bouts of morning sickness convinced me this pregnancy would unfold as Holden's had. I loved the tiny vibration of potential.

But the second week of March, just a few weeks after the visit to the castle hospital and receiving Holden's prescription for Depakote, I miscarried for the third time. During an early-morning writing session at my kitchen counter, I felt a cramp deep in my pelvis that made me drop my pen. I stumbled to the bathroom off our bedroom, slid my underwear down, and saw blood. My knees softened, and I slumped onto the toilet seat.

This time, I knew the pattern—and the pattern knew me. It cleaved something. My invisible tether to reality or control or rationality—sliced by this knowing—disappeared. The third miscarriage: pleading with God to reverse it, my sobs bouncing off the walls of the bathroom; calling my mother, asking her why God hated me, begging her to tell me what I'd done to deserve this; being coaxed out of bed by Abel (how had I gotten there? how long had I been there, bleeding?); seeing my uterus on the hospital's ultrasound screen, so still and so quiet. The technician said that the fetus had stopped growing three weeks earlier. When she called it a *missed miscarriage*, I remember Abel squeezing my hand. *Missed miscarriage.* How could I have missed it? How could I have not known?[2]

Before experiencing multiple miscarriages, I didn't perceive my body as something that could be so unknown, so confusing, and so unpredictable. Perhaps one of the qualities of a liminal space is not knowing when you're in one. In miscarriage, my body crossed between pregnant and not pregnant—two states of being that had seemed distinct. I remember wondering, as I left the clinic after the first miscarriage, whether the embryo was still there. For two days I didn't know, until bloodwork revealed *not pregnant*. The second time it took a physical examination. The third time, an ultrasound showed I'd lived in a liminal space for weeks—unknowing.

Unknowing felt so painful, and I wanted a reason for the pattern of miscarriage. So I blamed myself: I was defective. My body was supposed to give birth. That's what I saw in my community, in my family, in my friend groups. No one I knew had more than one miscarriage. At the third, I moved into the recurrent miscarriage category—shared by a mere percent of couples.[3] Even though I couldn't see the defect or explain the imperfection, with this miscarriage I moved from normal to abnormal. My body was defective. I was defective.

Defective sounded from the pen's zip when I signed the paperwork consenting to dilation and curettage (D&C)—a surgery I'd chosen rather than letting the fetus pass on its own; the thought of more bleeding terrified me. *Defective* bubbled up when the nurse handed me a hospital gown and demanded I remove my contact lenses. *Defective* passed through my mind as they wheeled me to the surgical room. It was the word I counted backward from into unconsciousness.

In the surgical room, the doctor took twenty minutes to scrape out my uterus. I woke groggy. A nurse drifted in and out and then hovered at the foot of my bed. Abel appeared. Then I was home. I found Holden on the cusp of sleep, and so I snuggled into his bed while he drifted off. *Be thankful for the child you have,* I thought as I studied Holden sleeping. I felt a swell of gratitude even as I mourned that sacred tissue lost to me, that twist of Abel's DNA with mine. It was the thought I'd given flesh, a container for my love, a room to be prepared. A hunger unsatisfied.

* * *

Rosemarie Garland-Thomson's work describes disability as both a social category and a social movement. In books, articles, and lectures, she explains how a person can move into disability through illness, injury, and aging. "Since most of us are not born into disability but enter into it as we travel through life," she writes, "we don't get acculturated" the way most of us do with other identity categories, such as race or gender. She urges her readers to prepare for disability rather than flee from it: "Clearly, the border between 'us' and 'them' is fragile."[4]

Before I encountered Garland-Thomson's work—over a decade after the third miscarriage—I embraced the dichotomies of us/them, able/disabled. Even though I understood gender and sexuality as fluid, disability seemed fixed. One is either disabled or one isn't, I thought; disability is a claim one makes or doesn't. But as I sat with Garland-Thomson's words, I imagined a body moving across a line, back and forth. I recognized the blur this back-and-forth movement creates—the blur that erases rigid boundaries, the blur of the liminal space. The liminal space of miscarriage.

After the third miscarriage, I explored miscarriage as liminal in poetry. In the book that became *Bluewords Greening*, I wrote poems articulating the space between knowing one is pregnant and learning one is no longer pregnant. And I'm not the only one to describe miscarriage in this way. In "The Event That Was Nothing: Miscarriage as a Liminal Event," Alison Reiheld argues that despite the frequent occurrence of miscarriage, silence and taboo cloak this phenomenon, and due to under-theorization, miscarriage gets "enrolled in larger debates over women's reproduction." Reiheld writes: "To truly understand why miscarriage is so taboo and to fully grasp the identity disruption that miscarriage poses, as well as to later understand how it becomes enrolled in social debates which are not really about miscarriage, we must first understand miscarriage as a liminal event."[5] She illustrates this identity disruption with continuums that pull apart binaries, such as non-parent/parent, death/life, etc. My poetry illuminates these continuums.

But it was only the new understanding of disability as fluid, combined with Garland-Thomson's explanation of what disables people, that helped me realize—from my own embodied experience—recurrent miscarriage as disability. What disables people, Garland-Thomson argues, are not the physical, mental, and emotional differences people possess, but how these differences are "collectively imagined as defective."[6] And when difference becomes defect, stigma surrounds it.[7] A person whose *bodymind*—a word that points to the inseparable relationship between body and mind—is different must contend with the burden of whatever assumptions or stories stigma assigns.

When I layered these insights, I traced my sense of defect after that third miscarriage to the stories that surrounded me, to expectations about what my body should do, to the fantasy of what a perfect female body should do. I felt angry that, as a feminist, I'd analyzed so many ways dominant narratives shape me—but not this one. A decade later, adopting this new framework gave me a way to revise my self-blame and remove the idea that my body made me defective. More importantly, it helped me understand how one can transgress the lines of us/them, able/disabled, across time. My experience of recurrent miscarriage was an experience of disability.

* * *

Recurrent miscarriage was also practice for Holden's frequent movement across the blurred lines that divide typical from atypical, ill from well, able from disabled. But I didn't yet know that I would need to move with him as his parent and advocate in ways that required flexibility and reorientation. That spring, after the third miscarriage, Holden's April seizure on the interstate, and the epic seizure in May, I clung to my own version of rigidity. Fear kindled along its usual routes, expanding each run. Defectiveness circulated with anxiety, and I found myself perpetually sad. If Theresa's death had felt like a meteor crashing onto the surface of my life—sudden, shocking, scarring—the events of that spring felt like a series of tornadoes touching down in my backyard.

I'd coped with Theresa's death, in part, by writing. In the months afterward, I wrote a story about four tight-knit sisters whose names started with A. In the opening chapter, their father dies of a heart attack. I projected my grief into fiction to disguise myself. I was Alicia— pretty, popular, heartbroken. I filled notebook after notebook with house-design details, and Alicia's room was red. I stacked my feelings onto the page in word-bricks, the story structuring my grief, the sisters surrounding Alicia supporting her. My actual family and friends helped me grieve, too. Slowly the meteor cooled, and we lived next to the impact site.

As a child, writing helped me externalize pain. Even a fictional character could carry it—carry both my heartache and longing. In hindsight, it helped me feel less alone, despite my circle of support. Alicia had sisters, and these girls survived. My pain took shape next to their story and gave me a welcome space to explore my grief through narrative and metaphor.

Writing poems in response to my particular series of tornadoes helped me record and process emotions, but it didn't offer solutions: I wanted another child, and I wanted to keep Holden safe. Perhaps adding the power of knowledge to The Plan, however subconscious it was at the time, fuelled the illusion that I had some control over these outcomes. As summer unfolded, I doubled down on miscarriage and epilepsy research.

When Holden was at daycare or off with Abel, I'd sit at my usual spot in my kitchen, mug of tea in my hand, and read. Miscarriage felt the most urgent because I believed Holden's medication (increased again after the epic seizure in May) had reached a therapeutic level. I needed to decide whether we should continue to try to conceive or start the adoption process—or both. The day of the third miscarriage, Abel and I talked about our future for an hour between fits of tears. We both wanted another child, and we agreed on adoption to expand our family. His words assured me we were experiencing both pain and hope together.

From fertility specialist websites, I jotted down possible causes of miscarriage: endocrine problems, autoimmune disorders, chromosomal abnormalities. Sometimes I copied sections in my notebook, my left-hand smudging ink across the page when I wrote too much too fast. A few websites praised Jon Cohen's *Coming to Term: Uncovering the Truth About Miscarriage*. Cohen seemed well-suited to wade through the "myth, hype, and uncertainty"[8] that pervaded information about pregnancy loss: he was a science-focused journalist, and his wife had lost four pregnancies.

I tracked down the book and read it cover to cover. Cohen used data to explain the state of medical knowledge about miscarriage, eschewing jargon. Because so many factors must align to bring life to fruition, it seemed incredible that I'd even conceived and carried Holden to term.

Cohen attributed most miscarriages to chromosomal abnormality, arguing that 50 to 70 percent of miscarriages occurred for this reason; had the pregnancies come to term, the children would've died shortly after birth or very early in infancy. By selecting out the unviable pregnancies, Cohen implied, the body cleared the way so another pregnancy could occur.

Cohen's case studies sparked reflection for me, too. Some women who miscarried went on to expand their families; some didn't. I reacted with disbelief to the stories of women who kept trying after more than five miscarriages—I was sure another would pull my attention away from Holden and Abel. I was certain more would break me. And yet the significant amount of medical intervention many of the women submitted to convinced me that a doctor's insight might help.

The second week of June, four months after the third miscarriage, I saw a fertility specialist in Sioux Falls. He asked me questions about my health and educated me about miscarriage in general: sometimes the problem is with the mother's anatomy (not the case with me), and sometimes the problem is hormonal—the body isn't releasing the right hormones, or the right amount of them. He ordered an extensive panel of blood work. He also pointed out that because I'd experienced two different types of miscarriage—two very early ones and one missed miscarriage—he couldn't pinpoint a cause. Chromosomal abnormality was his best guess, too.

As I sat with a needle in my arm, filling vial after vial with blood, I wondered if the mechanism of the chromosomal tangle at conception was to blame for my miscarriages—a line of reasoning that still allowed me to blame myself. I wondered if the bloodwork would reveal anything new. I wondered if I'd ever stop feeling betrayed by my body. I wondered if I'd ever carry another child to term.

But I also sat with clarity. I longed for another baby, and I knew that even if the chromosomes didn't divide properly and the pregnancy continued, I would love a child with a disability. I could take the emotional risk of another miscarriage, too. So I grasped onto Cohen's statistic: 70 percent of women who had three miscarriages go on to have a successful fourth pregnancy without any medical intervention. I closed my eyes and pictured ten circles of ten stick women, colouring them pink. Then I turned thirty stick women grey to represent those who would have a fourth miscarriage. The pink overwhelmed me—seventy was so much more than thirty. I hung my hope on that statistic. My plan? Among the pink stick women, I turned one purple. That would be me.

* * *

During my spring and early summer research binge, I shared everything I'd learned with Abel, and he seemed bolstered by the research too. We'd try one more time. We didn't have to cycle through months of expectation. Mid-July, I woke up at 4:00 a.m. to rain pounding the windows and lightning brightening the bedroom. I counted the days since my last period and couldn't go back to sleep, so I peed on a stick, as I had so many times before. In just a minute, two lines appeared. Pregnant. I shook Abel awake with the news.

"Merry Christmas, happy birthday," he said, half asleep and smiling. "Congrats."

I curled up next to him, listening to the storm and making new summer plans.

The next day, the cycle of doctoring began. Between the fertility specialist and my family doctor, I scheduled blood draws and checkups. I drove down to Sioux Falls to pick up my progesterone prescription—a batch of 1.5-inch-long white tubes that looked like wax, slightly wider than a pencil, and inserted like a tampon—an insurance policy against the luteal-phase defect that interfered with implantation. At the clinic in Brookings, hormone tests detected a strong pregnancy and ruled out a thyroid problem.

I gathered tools to help me grapple with my excitement and fear. I started a diary, writing to the unfolding embryo: *I wrap up the secret that is you in the tinfoil of hormones the doctor prescribed to help keep you growing as the vegetables in my garden have—basil from seed, cilantro and thyme, butternut squash and pole beans, silverbeet and fennel. I have no control over them. I have no control over you, only to make sure the soil was in good condition for sowing.*

I tried not to compare my pregnancy symptoms to the last pregnancies (was I feeling nauseous enough? not enough?) but did anyway, and those comparisons sparked cycles of worry. I mapped out the pregnancy week by week on my calendar, circling the due date: March 14, 2011. My kids would be five years and two months apart, I thought. And then six weeks of maternity leave would take me right to the end of the semester. I felt lucky.

In August, an appointment with a high-risk OB/GYN bolstered my confidence. She pointed to the yolk sac on the four-dimensional ultrasound displaying vibrant shades of yellow and orange and called it "a good size." I could hear the rushrushrushrushrush of cardiac activity and see the thrum moving on the screen. In the car, Abel looked at me, beaming.

"Looks like we'll be a family of four," I said. And I believed it.

I believed Cohen's research, comforted by statistics and stories. I believed in science, anatomy and taxonomies, methods and precision. These beliefs worked like magic, like religion. I saw the fetus on a screen, and each day, I pictured it growing strong and healthy, cells into tissues into organs into baby. I imagined my womb, an avocado-shaped sac of spun gold, and inside it, light. I breathed my prayer into the light. Each day without blood in my underwear increased my confidence: just as the research implied, my desire and my body were aligned.

But like the other three, my body jettisoned that pregnancy too. On September 2, Abel and I dropped Holden off at daycare and headed to Sioux Falls for an end-of-first-trimester appointment. I'd hoped driving to a new place would feel positive and that the doctor I'd selected would bring new knowledge to the table.

As I peppered her with every pregnancy question I could summon, she worked to move the Doppler in place.

"Let's listen to Baby first," she said to deflect my anxiety. I tuned into silence as she moved the tool across my belly. "Sometimes Baby is situated in such a way that makes it tough to hear. Let's try an ultrasound," she said.

I was silent, and I was sweating. *There's not going to be a heartbeat,* I thought. The image appeared on the screen, still and soundless.

"I'm sorry," she said. "It's measuring about nine weeks." Another missed miscarriage.

The OB/GYN said *Baby*. I said *fetus* and *mine*, and I loved it all the same.[9]

* * *

The next day, Abel drove me back to Sioux Falls for a D&C. As I waited for the procedure, I grew aware of how acutely my knowledge betrayed me. *Defective* looped through my brain, stronger than before. I cupped my belly, thicker than usual. My breasts ached. *It's not what it looks like, not what it feels like,* I told myself. *It's not here.* I couldn't trust my senses; I still felt pregnant. I couldn't trust the expertise of the doctors. I couldn't trust the statistics. How had I ever believed? I couldn't even trust myself. The fourth miscarriage sunk me deeper into my internalized defectiveness.

The procedure took forty-five minutes—twice as long as the last one—to render my uterus empty. When I emerged from the post-D&C fog (I lost a lot of blood and barely remember the next three days), I wondered whether a conversation with the doctor would reveal anything new. But after a few days, I stopped caring and never went to a follow-up appointment. No information would change my new conviction: another loss would break me.

Chapter Four

INTERFERE:
to intervene without invitation

AFTER I RECOVERED PHYSICALLY FROM THE MISCARRIAGE, I tried to move through the grief. I closed the door on the room I'd kept as a nursery-in-progress—the room where I stored Holden's old crib, baby clothes, and toys. When sadness overwhelmed me, I'd walk past that door and right into Holden's cheerful bedroom. Packed with books, superheroes, puzzles, and board games, the white furniture seemed to glow against the brightly painted walls: robin's egg blue on top, asparagus green on bottom. In between ran a border of animals: lion, zebra, giraffe, and elephant. My mother, the queen of crafting before DIY was cool, fashioned those same animals out of wood and fabric to decorate the walls. Two feet high, they matched the animals on the border exactly. Holden loved to run his fingers across their different textures: vinyl, felt, burlap, fur. And he loved to climb up on the reading bench my dad had built for him on one of his rare visits, homebody that he is. We'd placed the bench beneath a large west-facing window. The sunlight through that window always lifted my mood.

That autumn, I sank into the routine of teaching. Advanced Creative Writing and Writing Poetry were among my assigned courses—ideal, I thought. School schedules, no matter if I was student or teacher, steadied me. Each semester brought new students who would learn to write their lives or shape narratives drawn from their imaginations—sometimes both. They delighted me. I wanted them to learn that writing could be discovery—to quote Laurel Richardson, "a way of finding out about yourself and your topic."[1] I wanted this tool to serve them as it had me for so many years.[2] Teaching still felt challenging, but after more than a decade in the classroom, I could scrap detailed lesson plans and teach extemporaneously on any given topic in my curriculum. Knowing something so thoroughly felt good when so many other aspects of my life confounded me.

It had been four months since Holden's epic seizure in May, and his behaviour had become odd. Perhaps the haze of recovery from the fourth miscarriage dulled my sharpness, but I began to notice instances of him ignoring me—or rather, not seeming to hear me. One evening, I asked Holden if he wanted ice cream. He turned away, as if the words evaporated into the air before reaching his ear. I pointed to the container: "It's chocolate chip!" Then he got excited. My four-year-old's going on fourteen, I thought as I reached into the freezer.

These moments of not hearing accumulated like slow rain, scattered drops saturating my awareness over days. As they happened more often, I wondered what caused them. Absence seizures? No—he looked conscious. Defiance? No—Holden pushed his boundaries to negotiate another cartoon or a few more minutes of play but never beyond limits. Absorbed in an activity? No—he didn't immerse himself in play so deeply that he tuned me out.

There was something else, too: reciting dialogue from movies and picture books. One afternoon, while we were driving to the grocery store, Holden began to recite a conversation between Mater and Lightning McQueen from the movie *Cars*.

"You're in love with Miss Sally. / No, I'm not. / Yes, you are. / No way. / Way."

"What movie is that from?" I asked.

"You're in love with Miss Sally. / No, I'm not. / Yes, you are. / No way. / Way," he repeated.

"Is it from *Cars*? Which characters are those?" I hoped to shape a conversation.

"Yes," he said, ignoring the second question.

I chalked those moments up to Holden's personality as a quirky child until these odd exchanges occurred more often. Another day, on the five-minute drive to preschool, we played our usual rhyming game.

"Bat rhymes with—" I began. I glanced in the rearview mirror. Tucked into his car seat, Holden looked at me.

"Mat!" he said.

"Right. M-A-T," I said. "Mat rhymes with—"

"Cat!"

"Right. C-A-T," I said.

"Cat, not a bird, not a mouse or a grouse ..." He switched to a book he adored, and this association pleased me.

"Yes. That's from *Skippyjon Jones*. What happens in that book?"

"Not a rat or a bat ..." He picked up where he'd left off, then mumbled something. "A Siamese cat!" he finally announced.

"Do you like that book, Holden?" He didn't reply. I looked again in the mirror. Then he blinked hard. "Hey. Earth to Holden. Do you like that book?"

"What?" he asked.

"Oh, nothing," I said, pulling into the parking lot. "We're at school." But that long blink.

When I asked Abel if he'd noticed it too, he said that he assumed Holden had inherited his talent for memorizing movies. But that didn't explain why Holden would repeat parts over and over. It didn't explain why he wouldn't answer my questions afterward. The behaviour mystified us both.

* * *

Drip. Drop. A drizzle, not a deluge. Sometimes it takes time for the brain to recognize patterns among moments of observation; sometimes it takes a jolt of pressure for the floodgates of understanding to open.

I was prepping dinner, gathering ingredients from the pantry and refrigerator, when Holden walked over from the living room.

"Water!" He reached up, grabbing a tall glass. As he turned to take a sip, it slipped from his hands. Shards and ice cubes slid across the floor.

"Don't touch! I'll get the broom," I said. Holden looked at the watery mess, hands at his sides against his jeans. As I stepped away, he crouched down, reaching for the glass. "Don't touch. This is dangerous. It could cut you. Ouch!" So curious, I thought. I placed him on the barstool several steps from the mess. "I'll get you another glass of water in a second. Let me clean up this mess first." I cradled the largest shards in my palm to see how much of the glass had broken into smaller pieces. I wanted to account for all of it. Holden hopped down from the stool and walked toward me.

"Water!" He stepped forward. I grabbed the cabinet with my hand, blocking his legs. He pushed against my arm, plunging himself toward the floor. He acted as if a piñata had burst, as if the pieces of glass were candy.

Just in case he decided to treat my arm like a limbo bar, I scooted between him and the mess. That triggered something. Holden began to cry, then screamed something unintelligible. *What the hell? What's wrong with him?* I thought. Then I imagined his tender feet cut up and bleeding, slivers of glass wedged in his heels. A trip to the ER. Stitches. My anger softened.

"Calm down," I said. "I'll get you another glass. I'll get you more." As I cranked around to pitch the pieces into the garbage can, Holden jumped onto my back and clung, shoving his foot into my ribs. His insistence and intensity stunned me.

With Holden on my back and with one more barehanded sweep, I got most of the shards into the garbage. Then I placed Holden on the stool again and poured him a new glass of water. As he sipped, the redness of his face disappeared. Then he took two long gulps, put the cup down, and jumped off the stool. He turned from the mess and ran. I heard a toy bin slide off the shelf in his room. *He's playing now,* I thought. I grabbed the broom to finish cleaning.

As soon as the last bits hit the bin, I sat down on the stool Holden had vacated and took a deep breath. I was wiped out. As I exhaled, the storm clouds opened. *Something's not right, something's not right* pulsed in my brain, sharp and sparkly, and a vague sense shifted to conviction. Holden's fierce obsession with that glass was not normal. These moments of not hearing weren't normal. My child wasn't normal.

* * *

Tanya Titchkosky notes that "*normal is a referential system of sense making* and not a natural or pregiven conditions of existence."[3] In her entry for the book *Keywords in Disability Studies*, she points out the fluidity of normalcy—how what constitutes normal changes with time and context. She argues that the power of normalcy rests in its relationship to abnormality; normal becomes a "position from which people deem other people to be lacking, different, dysfunctional, deformed, impaired, inadequate, invalid."[4]

Normal and abnormal create a binary, and these days, binaries unsettle me. In their rigidity, their either/or-ness, they eclipse possibility and precision. When binaries like gender and sexuality become undone, their spectrums multiply with language and theories and narratives. And I've witnessed the power of naming the once-liminal spaces—of articulating thresholds. What happens when *normal / not normal* is pressed in similar ways? Undoing the power of a word like *normal*—a word that serves to exclude, deny, sort, and stigmatize—could be achieved by chipping away at its boundary.

But at the time of the broken-glass incident, *normal / not normal* seemed logical, natural, fixed. By reaching for shards of glass and by not always seeming to hear me, Holden moved beyond the boundary of *normal*—and questioning that move held no fascination. Had I understood the liminal space in which I stood with my son, I might have used more precise and helpful language to describe what I'd observed. Instead, I circled back to *not normal, not normal, not normal.*[5]

Over the next few weeks, three questions flooded my thoughts: What is normal for an (almost) five-year-old? What is normal for a child with epilepsy? What is normal for a child taking Depakote?[6] I asked my friends who were parents about whether they'd seen such big, dramatic episodes from their children. The broken-glass incident had been the most puzzling, but Holden had also melted down when he opened a nearly empty jar of applesauce and when I suggested that we read a book he didn't like at bedtime. Saying no to candy at the grocery store summoned tantrums. Most of my friends agreed that the frequency of this behaviour warranted concern, and nowhere in my research on epilepsy did I find this kind of behaviour discussed. More research on the side effects of Depakote (anxiety, agitation, insomnia, irritability, confusion, aggression) gave me pause, however. Could that be the root of these issues? I observed Holden, hoping my new knowledge of Depakote's side effects might help me identify a pattern. Did the behaviours happen in relationship to when he took his medication? I didn't find anything. The *not hearing* episodes continued with no apparent context, and his behaviour remained odd. When I learned that side effects from medications usually happen right away, not nine months down the road, I ruled that out as a cause.

After sorting through these thoughts for a couple of weeks, I understood that these behaviours weren't normal for Holden. In the referential system of my son, not hearing and erratic irritability didn't square with what I knew about the way he interacted, the way he experienced the world. And the broken-glass incident underscored that this change could be dangerous—as dangerous as a seizure. He would've put glass into his mouth if he'd reached it.

I conferred with one of Dr. Porter's nurses on the phone and told her about the changes in Holden. Could more testing be done? She suggested a twenty-four-hour video EEG to check on seizure activity. "The four-hour one he had in February might not have given Dr. Porter the whole picture," she said. I wondered, albeit briefly, why Dr. Porter hadn't wanted the whole picture at the beginning.[7]

* * *

Two weeks later, Holden was admitted to the children's hospital in Sioux Falls for the overnight video EEG. The procedure began with Holden sitting calmly in a chair for over an hour while a technician wired him up.

"You'll feel this electrode, now, on your skin." The tech pressed a plastic-covered metal disk to his scalp. Holden felt the result with his fingertips. "Didn't hurt, right?" she asked. Holden shook his head no. "Good. Touch it gently! It has to stay on until tomorrow."

"I'll be careful," Holden said. He stretched and shifted in his chair from time to time but otherwise didn't complain as the tech glued on the dozen or so button-sized electrodes. When finished, she wound gauze around his head and taped over it to create a cap. "This is so you won't accidentally pick at them in your sleep," she said to Holden, but looked at me, smiling. "I'll take them off tomorrow."

"Okay," Holden said. "Can I go to the bathroom now?"

"Sure." The tech manoeuvred the video equipment and all the wires so he didn't trip. The camera stayed outside the bathroom, and the cords were just long enough to allow him privacy to do his business. As I stood to help, the tech turned to me and said, "Just let the nurse know if you need anything—day or night." She waved goodbye and closed the door.

An EEG records the series of brain waves (patterns of normal or abnormal brain activity) as traces on software so a computer can save the data and, if needed, print it. Despite the video camera, which records visual data that can accompany a seizure, the tech tasked me to write down any suspicious seizure activity in a notebook so that Dr. Porter could scrutinize that part of the EEG in particular. These directions frustrated me, though. I couldn't distinguish between an absence seizure and spacing out; I wanted the twenty-four-hour video EEG to do so. Seeing a seizure or tracking times where seizures didn't exist—seizure or not seizure—should be simple with electrodes on his head, I'd thought. Now I see how easily I accepted the binaries that medicine presented to me. Flung out from *normal* and yet still feeling its pull, it felt logical to expect experts and their tests to resolve all these episodes of *not hearing*, to explain the meltdowns, and to put these in the context of epilepsy. It made sense that they would be the ones to restore Holden to normalcy.

Two months shy of five years old, Holden's body spanned a quarter of the hospital bed. He seemed to shrink into it, his bottom tucked into the bed's bend, the back raised up. Cross-legged, he used a *Kindergarten BOOTCAMP* box as a lap desk. He gripped a blue marker with his right hand, the exact grasp his preschool teachers modelled, and traced "b"—down to the line, up a bit, half circle—on the wipe-away sheet. Every minute or so, he paused to scratch his neck just below the gauze-and-tape cap, which made his head look wounded. He seemed to have fun writing his ABCs on the sheets with markers, a far cry from the grainy paper I'd ripped to shreds as a third grader who'd failed handwriting. It would be a few years before schools tested Holden on these concepts, but I was happy to see him learning so much so early.

Holden seemed on track for reading, and it brought me joy to think books would be a passion for us both. What's more normal than a parent wanting to connect with their child over a beloved activity? It seemed as if I'd always known how to read. By third grade, I'd read all the books that had piqued my interest in the primary school section of the library, so the librarian offered me books from the middle-school section. I chose books like *A Tree Grows in Brooklyn* and *Are You There God? It's Me, Margaret*. Books launched me into new worlds, and books fed my curiosity. Books meant an escape from family tensions, and books meant deepening my understanding of grief. In sixth grade, after Theresa's death, I needed both escape and solace. Books were sources of knowledge that made me happy, and I wanted them to work the same way for Holden. As I watched him practise his letters, I wondered what his first self-read book would be and which ones he'd love as he grew up.

After twenty minutes of *BOOTCAMP*, I cued up cartoons on the Disney Channel. Then I settled into the futon, which would transform into my bed that night, and watched Holden holler, "Toodles! Oh, Toodles!" just as Mickey did on *Mickey Mouse Clubhouse*. A magic bag appeared, and Mickey asked the audience to pick the right tool to solve his problem. Holden always ventured a guess, and he always giggled at Pluto.

Once I noticed him gazing between me and the TV—did he spot a contrail in the sky, or was he having a seizure?—so I wrote it down. Another time he gazed out the door for a few seconds. He asked to get up once, so I gathered the cords trailing down his back and we tiptoed, scissor-stepped, and skipped around the room to stretch our legs. Otherwise, the whole event was uneventful. The nurses brought meals, and the techs checked on him regularly. Abel drove down after work and relieved me so that I could walk around the hospital. He kissed Holden goodbye when it was time for bed. The pullout futon slept only one, and Abel didn't want to take more time off work than he had to.

The next morning, the tech came back and helped Holden perform two tests designed to elicit seizures: the pinwheel test and the strobe-light test. The first involved Holden blowing on a pinwheel for five minutes, which mimicked hyperventilation to trigger seizures. Holden smiled at the pinwheel and did his best to blow as hard as he could; I cheered him on when he got tired or bored. I didn't notice any visible seizures. During the strobe-light test, we again encouraged Holden to keep his eyes open as the light flashed in his face, and again, no seizures.

After the tech removed the electrodes, I helped Holden soap up in the shower, and he let me comb through his glue-flecked hair with minimal fuss. Just as the tech began to walk out, I thanked her and asked if she'd seen any seizures on the EEG. Unfortunately, she wasn't allowed to interpret the EEG for patients, but she assured me that Dr. Porter would call soon with the results.

* * *

The following weekend, Abel and I left Holden in the care of good family friends in Minnesota so we could attend a conference sponsored by the Epilepsy Foundation of Minnesota, an organization that serves people with epilepsy and raises awareness of seizure disorders for the general public. I soaked up information at talks titled "The Whole Child: Conditions Associated with Pediatric Epilepsy," "Ketogenic Diet and Management Considerations," and "Enhancing Academic Success: A Neuropsychological Perspective." In light of the EEG—but not yet having results—I was eager to learn something about epilepsy and behaviour, but no one addressed Holden's issues, and the presenters rarely left time for questions.

At the evening keynote on the differences between generic and brand-name medications, Abel and I sat down at a table set with cloth napkins and multiple forks per place setting. We—and the hundred or so other attendees—had paid to attend this conference, but it was a reasonable fee, so this elegance surprised me. Behind the main podium, a screen featured a photo of a young man in his twenties—the same dark hair as Holden, a similar winning grin. This young man had glasses, though, and hazel eyes. He appeared to have a zest for life—that same charisma I saw in photos of Theresa. Under the photo: *Jacob Ronald Knapp: 08/05/86–03/02/09. Cause of death: SUDEP.* My appetite vanished. What was SUDEP?

The emcee for the evening took the stage and welcomed everyone. Then he thanked the guests of honour, the Knapp family. The Knapps had raised over $23,000 for SUDEP research in honour of their son, Jake, who had died the year before while in his final semester at Columbia College. "When his parents were told, they had no idea what SUDEP was," the emcee said. "SUDEP, or Sudden Unexpected (or Unexplained) Death in Epilepsy, occurs when someone with diagnosed epilepsy passes away without any other cause."[8]

My stomach lurched and heaved. For a second, I thought I might vomit at the table. Every cell rebelled against this knowledge; it felt like a virus, an invader. No one had told me about this possibility. And I'd missed it in my research. How could I not have known about this?

The emcee described SUDEP as something that happened during sleep, so no one observed the victims at the time of death. Risk factors included age—usually between 20 and 40—and uncontrolled seizures. He said that each year, one in a thousand people with epilepsy died from SUDEP.

The Knapps stood up and acknowledged the applause. Once, the rarity of SUDEP would've rendered the statistic meaningless to me, but after the miscarriages, statistics meant real—not remote—possibility. I fought my impulse to run up and hug the parents of Jake Knapp. To run up and shake them for answers. To run up and cry with them. I imagined Jake's roommate finding him dead in bed, then replayed that scene with his girlfriend finding him. Then I imagined the hundreds of parents and loved ones who had woken up one day to find their beloved dead in bed. I imagined Holden at my friend's house. I wanted to call her and scream, *Stay vigilant. Watch him all night long. Don't sleep.* Instead, I texted her. She texted back. He was fine and having a great time.

The keynote speaker explained that when a coating or dye is added to a drug, it can influence the drug's absorption in the body. As a result, sometimes a switch between brand names and generics (or vice versa) can lead to breakthrough seizures—when someone whose seizures are usually controlled by medication has a seizure. I know this only from the few notes I took to force myself to pay attention and stop obsessing about Holden's risk factors.

As Abel and I walked to our room, tears streamed down my face. "Had you heard of SUDEP before?" I asked.

"No." His voice was steady and sober. I stifled a sob.

"What should we do?"

"Learn more. But right now, it doesn't seem like there's anything we can really do."

Unexpected. Unexplained. Even experts couldn't explain or expect; even experts didn't know. If they didn't know, how could I? If they didn't have solutions for how to keep people alive, how could I keep Holden safe?

The next morning, Abel went to two sessions before excusing himself. "I'm going to sit out awhile," he said. "There's been a lot of information."

I nodded and grabbed my notebook off the table we'd been sharing. For a moment I thought about pressing him to come with me. I understood this amount of information took time to absorb, and I knew that Abel and I tended to process information differently. I liked to talk about it; he preferred to think about things alone. At the same time, we lived four hours away in a rural area and didn't have easy access to experts. We still had so much to learn in order to keep Holden safe.

But I remembered other times when I'd pressed Abel to join me at some activity only to regret it. Once, I'd begged him to come with Holden and me to the Fourth of July parade in Brookings, even though he said no at first. At the parade, Abel stood four feet behind us, headphones on. He listened to music as Holden squealed in delight when the bands marched by and people threw candy from floats. I'd felt a bit embarrassed that he didn't seem to want to interact with us. After a few instances like this, I knew not to press. Afraid to confront Abel about joining me for more education, I grabbed the schedule and made plans to meet him when the conference was over.

* * *

The field of medicine invests in normalcy—and, in many ways, *invents* normalcy. I remember the first time I saw a height-and-weight chart at the doctor's office. I was a 125-pound teenager, and according to the chart, I was on the upper end of a normal weight range. Achieving a more average weight became my goal. I counted calories obsessively; one day I fasted and passed out in the shower. Thirty-odd years later, I still grapple with the shape of my body, even though I know how to critique messages about health and fitness. And yet that chart—that seemingly objective measurement—seemed so clear, so unbiased.

When I recall this period of unfolding epilepsy, I'm struck by the deep dive I took into the medicalization of disability without even knowing it. I pinned my hopes on the overnight EEG to yield immediate answers, and attended a conference where most of the presentations centred on medication and interventions—I had no other language, no other model, from which to stand in relationship to epilepsy. I was fully committed to medicine solving Holden's seizure disorder. Believing that knowledge is power meant that those with the most knowledge—medical professionals—had the answers, but I didn't consider that they also wielded the power to shape how I thought about epilepsy and my relationship to it as Holden's mom.

Under the medical model of disability, the medical establishment invests in curing, fixing, and restoring; suffering patients become normal again, or as normal as possible. Nowhere was I encouraged to think about barriers Holden might face, what social forces could disable him, or how having epilepsy might exclude him from typical childhood experiences. No one helped me explore the stigma of epilepsy. And despite my passion for learning and culture, not once did I look into the history of epilepsy and the academic analyses of seizure disorders. I didn't even know they existed. And in my rural town, these narratives were nearly invisible.

My meeting with Dr. Porter to discuss Holden's overnight EEG results reinforced my deep dive into the medical model, even as it pointed to a new, more precise degree of *not normal.*

* * *

In her book-lined office, Dr. Porter put down the pen in her right hand.

"Before I explain the results," she said, "I will show you the EEG data itself." She unfolded a long sheet of paper and pushed her hair behind her ear. As I attempted to understand what I was seeing, a sense of exhaustion flooded me. I wished Abel had taken the day off to accompany me, but the appointment was six weeks after the EEG, and Dr. Porter's office didn't offer many choices for time slots. My Friday afternoons were more flexible.

"Holden's brain waves are abnormal, as one would expect in a child with epilepsy," she said, arranging the printout. I expected to see black-threaded zigzags like the kind my mother's sewing machine made on fabric; instead, I saw erratic lines like a child's scribbles the first time holding a pen. "Here are the slow waves and spikes when he's sleeping." She pointed with her pen for emphasis. I followed the data with my eyes. Seismic activity. Here, here, and there. And there. Then, not here or there. I tried to understand. Did height matter? Space between the pointed tops? Were there patterns?

Dr. Porter launched into an explanation. I gripped my pen so hard my fingers started to tingle. I wrote down phrases: "one spike per minute when he's sleeping," "epileptiform abnormalities." But even a few words in medical jargon slowed me down as I tried to define them; I wasn't hearing everything she said.

I looked back at the printout, wondering how to read it. As I followed the lines, they started to move like a musical score drawn through a machine. The spikes and waves merged. I noted Dr. Porter's serious tone, the lack of animation in her speech. I wrote down "trouble sleeping, track his learning, look for problems."

A catalogue of Holden's learning appeared in my mind. A month before his second birthday, he'd learned the words eyes, please, careful, peas, nose, up, Mommy, Daddy, shoes, blocks, book, one-two-three, puppy, and ball. He'd learned animal sounds, too: moo, hoo-hoo (owl), hiss (snake), meow, and woof. Two days after his second birthday, he spoke his first combination of words, "puppy hug." Between the ages of two and four, he learned his ABCs and the sounds those letters make. He even learned a few words in Spanish. He took turns in conversations.

He counted. He added one plus one. He learned to swim, socialize, and play....

"Do you have questions?" Dr. Porter asked.

Somehow, I'd been in her office for forty-five minutes. The questions existed in syllables and sounds—grunts, coos, moans. I blinked. My hand was still poised to take notes. I sat up straighter in my chair. Questions? I had no words.

"Umm," I said. I'd made a mental note to ask a question before the meeting. "Oh. I remember. Those tests the tech did with Holden—the pinwheel, the strobe lights."

"He's not sensitive to flashing lights," Dr. Porter said. "And the other test didn't reveal anything useful."

"What about the places I noted where I may have seen seizure activity?"

"No. Those weren't seizures," she said. "Any other questions?" The tone of her voice signalled that we were in a new category, that *not normal* meant something else now. I glanced back at the printout, but it didn't summon any questions.

"No," I said. "Not now." I was intellectually shocked. My body sat, breathed, and looked attentive, but my mind had spun so fast it lost its centre.

I left her office with a prescription for Valium—for Holden, not me. It would work with the Depakote, she'd said. I was halfway to my car when thinking resumed. I hadn't noticed any sleep problems, so why did she assume he was having them? Perhaps if he developed poor-quality sleep it could lead to learning problems? And what had she said about an epilepsy syndrome? That the data didn't fit all the criteria, so she didn't want to diagnose him with it. On the drive home, I thought about how odd this seemed. Valium felt like a big solution to an anticipated problem that he didn't fit all the criteria for. Was this a space on the spectrum of normal/not normal that the expert could point to but not name?

I puzzled over her recommendation that we anticipate learning problems. Later that night, after reporting the appointment to Abel, I looked through Holden's scrapbooks where I'd documented his learning.

Just as I'd thought, Holden had always met learning milestones on schedule. Photos at two months: Holden in his *Very Hungry Caterpillar* sleeper, cooing at me behind the camera (eye contact); Holden's head turned to look at his dad (response to sounds). Photos at four months: Holden reaching for toys dangling above him (a second later he rolls over); Holden smiling at grandmother (interaction). Photos at six months: Holden playing catch with another child (gross motor skills); Holden pointing at the windsocks on the Santa Monica Pier, smiling (laughing); Holden pounding the keys on his baby piano and "singing" (babbling). Photos at nine months: taking Uncle T.J.'s hat on and off, on and off (gross motor skills); Holden flipping through books and babbling the words (language-specific sounds). When Holden began daycare after his first birthday, I documented his learning accomplishments on paper.

As Holden and I settled down on his bed to read, that erratic EEG superimposed itself on the book cover, spikes and waves blurring the letters. Everything I'd read about epilepsy argued that seizures didn't affect cognitive functioning, so I had no idea why they might cause learning problems. I blinked hard, pushing that vision away. Then I kissed Holden on the head and began to read: "Llama llama red pajama reads a story with his mama." Holden looked up at me and smiled. "I love this book, Mommy."

Chapter Five

INTERNECINE: destructive to both sides in a conflict

AFTER HOLDEN'S EPIC SEIZURE IN MAY, DR. PORTER INCREASED his Depakote level again, and with the summer unfolding without another seizure, my confidence grew that we'd reached a therapeutic level—a level at which the medication would be effective without causing adverse side effects. Yet even after I pulled open the capsule of Depakote and sprinkled it in Holden's pudding or applesauce each morning and night, I often woke up at 2:00 a.m. with an urgent need to check on him. I kept the thermometer handy so I could take his temperature at random times to see if he was running a low fever that might spike later. With any sneeze, cough, or runny nose, I took him to the doctor's office for evaluation. I kept the emergency medication in the same place at home and in my purse every time I headed out. This vigilance was planned, outlined, time-stamped.

And yet, alongside this outer layer of urgent attention emerged an inner one—an internal pressure. It threaded itself around my heart, around my lungs, between the muscles in my limbs, and along my spine. Then the pressure pulled, tightening. A barely perceptible shift but an increase of visceral tension. Later, I'd realize that the tension never loosened, only compounded over time. The odd behaviour, the not-quite-diagnosis, and the additional prescription for Valium only heightened my sense that Holden's well-being was contingent upon my vigilance.

Years after, when I felt the layer of urgent attention tightening, a friend shared the signs of high-functioning anxiety, and I began to connect some of my experiences.[1] High-functioning anxiety is an informal way to describe someone who experiences anxiety and yet still achieves success in daily life activities; they appear to others as ambitious, perfectionistic, and organized, but they feel overwhelmed, burned out, and full of self-doubt. On the outside, a person who functions well with anxiety may appear calm but internally fears failure. When I recognized myself in this description, I wondered if anxiety was my default mode, so much so that I didn't recognize other ways to exist, other ways to move through the world. Perhaps my family's grief over Theresa's death and my father's alcoholism seeded my anxiety as a child. Perhaps it was simply my personality. Perhaps I'd lived so long with pressure that I'd accepted the way it shaped me. Perhaps I'd always discounted pressure because it felt *normal*.

When I reflect on the events of 2011, I see how the increasing vigilance of parenting Holden and the dissolution of my marriage only added to my grief-wracked brain. I understand how anxiety can affect certain contexts but not others, how it can shut a person down at times and yet could fuel one's motivation at others. My version of anxiety fuelled The Plan for over two decades, but I'm sure it cost me many missed opportunities for fun and pleasure and erased the balance I'd aimed to achieve.

And so, despite all the logical reasons I might've let go of my wish for another child, I pursued it. I was meant to be someone else's mom. It was part of The Plan, but also the twisted tether of hope I grasped onto when pulling myself through the emotional aftermath of the miscarriages. Pursuit offered balm for my grief. Several months after my fourth miscarriage, I returned in earnest to the research I'd casually begun the summer before: adoption.

Stability is an easy pane to fracture when the pressure of one's own personality already applies so much stress.

* * *

In the margins of the day, I skimmed websites and tracked down resources about traditional adoption, interracial adoption, transnational adoption, and foster-to-adopt programs. If I learned about a philosophical argument for or against a particular kind of adoption or practical advice to plan out the endeavour, I shared it with Abel during dinner or as we cleaned up the kitchen. I hoped to hear, "Let's move forward on that," or "I agree, I'm in." Instead, he dodged by changing the subject. If Holden interrupted with "I want water" or "Where's my book?" distraction had the same effect. If we shifted to topics regarding the news or workplace drama, adoption disappeared. By the time Holden went to bed and Abel queued up the latest binge-worthy show, I was too exhausted to talk.

Considering that Abel needed to think about it on his own first, I tried an indirect method. I emailed him some book titles with the note, "Let's read the one about transracial adoption together." I hoped he'd order one of the books for both of us. He never replied, and no book arrived. Perhaps he was annoyed—frustrated, even—by my research-and-action mode. Perhaps he couldn't explain that adoption felt too abstract. Perhaps Holden's epilepsy diagnosis caused mental noise so loud that he couldn't make room to sort out the complex layers of adoption. I often felt overwhelmed, but, congruent with my personality, I still pushed forward.

One evening, when we were visiting my parents in Des Moines, we left Holden with them for a date night. By the time our food arrived, we'd covered our usual topics: a funny skit on *Saturday Night Live*, the latest news in our extended family, the political landscape. As we took our first bites, I brought up adoption; over kofta and korma, the subject couldn't disappear.[2]

"Let's talk about adopting a baby," I said. "I think it's time."

Abel sat back and looked down at his plate. "Have you thought about it? There are so many routes. We could add to our already ethnically mixed family. You've always said people from the Dominican Republic are a mix of African, Taíno, and Spanish peoples." I smiled at him.

He smiled back and nodded but said nothing. It wasn't race that tripped him up, I thought, but something else. I switched lines of argument.

"It's a lot of work to get this underway," I said. "We'd have to organize our finances. It can cost $25,000 for private adoption, which can include legal fees and health care for the birth mother. Plus, there are applications to fill out, even a scrapbook to introduce us to prospective birth mothers," I said. I told him about my friend's experience with adoption, how her husband had hesitated. She'd pieced together his background information from stories he'd told her; he just signed off. "As soon as their son came home, he was so grateful that she'd pushed," I said. "Of course, that's not ideal. I'd prefer to do it together, like the way we planned our wedding."

Abel listened, but he didn't ask questions or offer any insight. I stopped talking and looked at him, expectant. I didn't want the night to end in stone-faced impasse. He didn't seem angry, just ambivalent.

After a long pause, we each spooned more rice onto our plates and ate awhile in silence. Was I being unrealistic? Too pushy?

"Take a few weeks to think about this," I said, wanting to signal my patience. "Then let me know, because it takes work. Not like the getting pregnant part didn't take work," I said, winking, "but you know—that's more fun than paperwork."

He smiled. And even though I'd hoped he'd ask questions or discuss his fears or mention some preferences for a way to tackle this opportunity, the conversation dissolved there. The rest of the evening stayed superficial and strained, but even that awkwardness disappeared the next day. I focused on being optimistic so he could have time to reflect.

About a month later, I received his answer—firm and resolute. I'd been mulling adoption over in the shower. It could take years, and my planning mode put pressure on the practical: paperwork, timelines, finances. I dried off and got dressed. I couldn't start any of that without Abel's consent. When I yanked a comb through my hair and slammed it back on the shelf next to disposable razors and a bar of soap, I realized the extent of my frustration. When Abel had held me after the third miscarriage, he promised to adopt if we couldn't have another biologically.

On the ride home after the fourth miscarriage, he said adoption would be the way we'd go. We needed to act.

I walked out of the bathroom and saw him standing at the end of the hallway in his kickboxing pants and running shoes, poised to walk up the stairs.

"Hey," I said. "I really need to know about this adoption thing. Do you want to move forward with it or not? If so, we need to sit down and work on the application." He paused. He drew himself up to his full five feet ten inches and turned his head to me. His eyes narrowed. He said nothing.

"Don't you want another child?" I asked. "You said before that you did."

"I did," he said. "But it just doesn't seem to be in the cards for us to have another."

"I know." I felt a wave of defectiveness, responsibility. "At least biologically. But that's why we can adopt. We just need to decide how."

"I know it would make you happy," he said. "But that isn't a good enough reason to bring another child into our family." His shoulders turned toward me, and he pushed his glasses up on his nose. He seemed to square off. "I've decided I don't want to."

"What do you mean, you don't want to?" I asked. My skin tightened around my face. I could feel my wet hair dripping onto my cheeks.

"I just don't," he said. "Adoption doesn't feel right anymore."

I stared at him as the air rushed out of me. I wanted to crawl across the seven feet that separated us and beg him to change his mind. I wanted to cry, *But I'm meant to be someone else's mom!* Instead, I worked to steady my voice and restrain my emotions. *Breathe in. Breathe out. Be reasonable,* I told myself. *You wanted him to be honest, didn't you?*

Reflecting on this later, I recognized a pattern. Abel processed his thoughts internally; he wouldn't engage with me until he'd made up his mind unequivocally. I talked, explored, conjectured, critiqued, questioned; he listened, then decided. And that decision held. Despite my disappointment and anger, I wanted to make space for his voice—for the fact that he'd asserted himself after so much silence.

"This might take a while for me to accept." My calm voice surprised me. I wanted to crumble to the floor.

"I know," he said. "I'm sorry." I believed him and dropped it that day.

Running errands in the car a few weeks later, though, I raised it again. I told him that I was ready to move on with our lives, but that I needed to know the reason behind his change of heart.

"I had four miscarriages, and I don't know why. Doctors couldn't tell me why. God isn't going to tell me why. But you—you've chosen to close this door and you—you can tell me why." My voice cracked with tears. I felt desperate for an answer; without one, I blamed my defectiveness, my unworthiness.

"I don't know why," he said.

Just didn't know? I wondered. Or couldn't tell me? Wouldn't tell me? All I needed was a reason, an emotion: *I feel overwhelmed,* or *It feels too hard.* Something. Anything. But, as with all the answers I sought from Abel, this one would arrive on his timeline.[3]

* * *

I coped with my disappointment by keeping busy. After all, wasn't I hard-working and ambitious? I filled my time with tasks and my mind with plans. And I fantasized about travel. Travel meant escape from the mounds of baby and toddler gear I needed to trash or sell or give away. Travel meant a reprieve from chores and meal prep. Travel meant an immersion in the sensory experience of a new place—food, music, people, stories. But travel also offered a way to focus on repairing my relationship with Abel and set the stage for how we'd function as a family of three. I pitched Ireland to Abel over dinner one night, and by the end of the conversation, he volunteered to research cheap flights and reasonably priced accommodations.

I didn't expect to encounter another manifestation of my anxiety. On our mid-May flight, the Aer Lingus plane had been in the air for an hour when I started rocking in my seat. At first it was slight, my bent head tapping the headrest in front of me. My chest moved forward, then my torso moved back. Forward, back. Then the pace quickened. Perhaps this trip wasn't a good idea, I thought. My claustrophobia hadn't been this bad before.

Abel queued up a movie for Holden and the story quickly absorbed him. I wasn't so easily distracted. My legs started to shake. I pushed my back into the chair—an illusion of more space—but still felt trapped. Sprinting down the aisle and flinging the door open at 37,000 feet seemed a reasonable way to cope with the pressure mounting in my body.

I looked at Holden, his headphones curled over his ears. He giggled and pointed at the screen. My panic pressed on, summoning a memory of Holden in the tub with vomit trickling from his nose. My heart shook its fist: *If he seized now, what could you do?* Keep him sleeping well; keep him eating well; reduce stress. I whispered my safety litany, but it failed to calm me—the trip had dismantled it. Air travel increased his risk of illness and thus lowered his seizure threshold. No doctor could be rushed onto the plane. Holden's sleep was already disrupted. I toggled between rational lines of thought and the non-rational belief that Holden could die because I wasn't controlling every factor in my power.

A trip to the washroom and a pleasant conversation with a flight attendant distracted me enough to calm down. She encouraged me to see my choice to travel despite my worries as courageous. As I dabbed the smeared mascara off my cheek and took my seat, I felt sure that I could endure the rest of the flight without another panic attack. Yet I also felt more fragile, my confidence in my coping compromised.

* * *

Had Holden's seizure disorder and my conversations with Abel taken a deeper psychological toll than I'd realized? Anxiety while flying felt familiar; I'd felt rumblings of airplane panic in my late twenties, the first time I flew after the World Trade Center fell in 2001. I chalked it up to the shock of watching planes fly into skyscrapers over and over again in the media. But when I calmed down from the panic on the Aer Lingus flight, I remembered that I'd felt a similar kind of fear-fuelled anxiety the month before—and not on an airplane. At a conference in Atlanta, I'd missed a call from Holden's school. With no message left, I speculated: maybe Holden had a high fever, and they couldn't get hold of Abel; maybe he had a seizure at preschool and had cracked his head open. The room shifted, tilted. I called back, but no one picked up. By the final ring, sweat was beading off my body. I imagined kicking off my heels and sprinting to South Dakota. Half an hour later, they called back—Holden just didn't feel well. This panic seemed to mean something else, but what?

In the decade since posing this question, I've sought insight from research. I found a smattering of medical scholars—doctors, psychologists, healthcare professionals—who have made formal inquiries into the mental health of parents of children with epilepsy and published their research in journals like *Epilepsy & Behavior*, *Epilepsy Research*, and *Epilepsia*. The articles I found list teams of researchers from around the world: China, Canada, Israel, the United Kingdom, and the United States. All note an increased rate of anxiety and depression in parents of children with epilepsy, most often in mothers. Chloe Jones and Colin Reilly, in a systematic review that looked at a variety of previously published studies, clearly established that "families of a child with epilepsy have been found to experience significantly more stress, anxiety, and restrictions in family life than other families."[4] These studies clarified what I experienced. Combining the danger that seizures posed with the vigilance required to keep them at bay made my increased panic seem more understandable, perhaps even logical. The gestalt of these studies comforted me with the knowledge that, around the world, parents were experiencing a similar emotional reality.

Yet some of the specific assertions the researchers made troubled me. Aynur Pekcanlar Akay et al. found that anxious mothers "failed to develop supportive and friendly relationships with their children."[5] R. Lv, L. Wu et al. argued that "An intact family environment is probably one of the most important protecting factors for a patient with epilepsy."[6] Chapieski et al. stated that "Parents' reaction to their child's medical condition may distort their interactions with their child and that, in turn, may interfere with normal social development."[7] I read these assertions as laced with judgment and blame, even if many of the same researchers indicated that help and resources should be provided for parents. Perhaps because I knew how rare help and resources could be, they left me uneasy. Despite the importance of naming the stressors and acknowledging the need to address them, I see the chasm between identifying stress and providing support to minimize it. And no studies I read made clear proposals for who should be responsible for providing said support.

The inventory forms these studies used to gather data left me dissatisfied, too. Many of the researchers asked parents about anxiety by requiring them to distill months—perhaps years—of experience into a series of questions answered by yes/no/maybe or mostly likely/least likely/not likely at all. I wondered what they might see if they asked for anecdotes, stories even. So much is lost without context, histories, layers of experience. What would they find if they asked parents to trace anxiety's trajectory across months? Years? Would they find what anxiety rents in the body? Would they determine how long it takes a body, or a life, or a marriage to shatter?[8]

* * *

For three days, we drank stout in several of Dublin's family-friendly pubs and feasted on fish and chips. Holden enjoyed the food and the stimulation of the city as we explored it in a stroller designed for travel. Then we hopped on a bus that took us south to Cork, where we toured the historic districts, before heading to Galway via the Ring of Kerry in a rental car. The pace of the trip slowed as we drove through the Lee River Valley. Walls of stone surrounded green meadows, and here and there sheep nibbled grass. Plants, animals, towns, landscapes—everything was saturated with colour and scent, texture and weather.

Holden seemed saturated by sleep. In the car on our way to Staigue Fort, he dozed despite a good night's sleep. I poked him when I saw something that I thought he'd enjoy.

"Hey Holden! Look at that sheep. Maybe it's Shaun the Sheep," I said, hoping a favourite animated character might interest him. Holden's drooping eyes sprang open for a few seconds but then shut again. I hoped our stop at the fort, built during the Iron Age, would excite him. We turned off the main artery and onto another road that seemed to divide a grove of trees. When it ended in a parking lot, we got out and stretched.

"Ready to run around a cool old fort?" I tried to coax Holden out of the car, but when he only yawned, I unbuckled his car seat and turned my back. "Piggyback ride?" I asked. He clambered on. As we approached the Celtic stone ring, open to the sky, I waited for him to wiggle down. I imagined him running toward the fort or rolling in the grass or placing his palm on a stack of stones. Instead, he put his head on my shoulder.

When I finally got him awake enough to stand, Abel took him by the hand and walked into the inner pocket of a wall, showing him how to explore. I could hear Abel's voice instructing him in an especially excited tone. Holden smiled at first, but then it faded, so we gave up and headed back to the car. As we drove toward our next stop, he stared out the window at Ireland's misted fields until he succumbed to sleep again.

Could I blame the medication? From January through March, Holden's behaviour had improved a bit, which I chalked up to the Valium's effect on his sleep. *By getting better sleep, he's able to control himself,* I thought. Our parent–teacher conference in April convinced me that Holden's learning was on track, his intellectual and social milestones met. Yet that same month his meltdowns—like the one with the broken glass—began to happen more frequently. Dr. Porter increased his dose of Valium based on a phone conversation. The high dose alarmed the pharmacist who filled the new prescription. "It'll surely knock him out at night," he said. "But you shouldn't see the side effects—drowsiness, slurred speech, and confusion—because the medicine should be through his system by morning."

Seeing the extent of Holden's daytime sleepiness on that trip convinced me that the increased dose wasn't working as intended. One hundred fifty-four days of Valium seemed excessive. Moments of not hearing were happening more frequently, too, but they were tangled with sleepiness—was it a sleep-saturated haze that kept him from concentrating or answering? Was it seizure activity? We seemed to be back at the beginning.

And he still cried and raged and refused. In Galway, walking around the town's eighteenth-century Eyre Square and boutiques within the Latin Quarter made us hungry. After we found a restaurant in the guidebook, Holden didn't want to walk anymore but got mad when I suggested he hop into the stroller. That should've been a clue.

We ducked into a pizza shop a few blocks away, the scent of garlic and tomatoes compounding my hunger.

"I don't want pizza," Holden said, loud enough for the men behind the counter to hear. "I want hamburgers." I hoped the clerk would forgive his rudeness, since cajoling him to apologize would make this worse.

"We chose this place, Holden. They make pizza here." Holden scowled. We ordered a few slices of plain cheese and took them upstairs to the dining area.

"I don't like this cheese." He picked up the oozing mozzarella with his index finger and thumb and pulled. The cheese slid onto the plate.

"Just eat the crust and sauce, then," I said. We ate in silence. When Holden finished, he popped up. As soon as he began to wander around the dining room, I sensed a meltdown or tantrum was imminent.

Like the clichéd train wreck one can see coming, Holden's meltdowns and tantrums took time to build, and I'd grown accustomed to my responses. Whereas other five-year-olds moved through meltdowns quickly, or a parent could step in and redirect the child, Holden couldn't see any other perspective at all, even one that would benefit him. Sometimes meltdowns and tantrums overlapped, but most of the time they were distinguishable. Both followed Holden's inability to get what he wanted or when his expectations were dashed, but meltdowns involved whining and real tears—as opposed to forced tears; his body slumped into a chair or onto the ground for five, six, sometimes even ten minutes. Tantrums involved yelling and insisting; often, he'd push a chair or a person standing next to him and stomp his feet. They, too, lasted a long time.

"I want Sprite," Holden said.

"You already had some," Abel said.

"Here, we're almost ready to go," I said. "Why don't you put your jacket on?" Instead, Holden tossed his water bottle onto the floor.

Abel grabbed the stroller, and I assembled our stuff as quickly as we could. I wanted to avoid a public meltdown. I often felt judged by others, as if my parenting flaws were responsible for his tantrums. I wanted to avoid the shock and disdain on the faces of other diners. We were struggling to get Holden down the narrow stairs in the stroller when, quite suddenly, he began to cry. Tears and tears and tears. Nothing could calm him.

"What's going on with him?" I asked. Abel's eyes met mine. Our gaze held for a minute; we were both clueless, still. It hurt to see our son so distraught, and it hurt to have an audience for it. But even more so, it hurt not to understand why this was happening in the first place.

* * *

Bright spots of togetherness juxtaposed with hazy spots of confusion comprised the rest of the trip. At the Cliffs of Moher, seven hundred feet above the Atlantic, Holden ran ahead of me on the wind-whipped path, but at least he felt energized enough to bounce up the steps of O'Brien's Tower, a lopped-off castle top placed at the cliff's highest point. He waved down at his dad below, who had declined the view from the tower with us. Along the Burren, Holden held my hand as we crept along the shale—thin panes of flagstone—peering into fissures to see how far down the cracks opened up the earth. He squealed with excitement when he found a snail's shell the size of a nickel and a surreal shade of blue. Even as we tiptoed on plates of slate-coloured rock, it moved under our heels. We felt it cracking. At various moments, Abel would turn to me with an expression of tenderness, and I'd wonder what he was thinking. Even though our conversations rested on surfaces—practical travel, entertaining Holden, Irish history—we hadn't fought, and there hadn't been any moments of tension-filled silence. Abel had surprised me with a few off-the-beaten-path stops on our itinerary that he knew I'd enjoy, which gave me hope. It meant he cared; perhaps it meant that he was trying to mend the rift between us that had appeared when he changed his mind about adoption.

Researchers who study parental anxiety note a prevalence of "marital discordance." Whether it stems from increased responsibility for treatments, fear of seizures, or constant vigilance, these changes affect a couple's interactions. "The chronic illness of children could change family roles, causing anger or guilt in the parents. Parents could become isolated from family and friends, which may limit the parents' ability to pursue their own interests," wrote the team of Aynur Pekcanlar Akay et al.[9] Add a shift in a child's behaviour, and rates of anxiety and depression increase. And because epilepsy and intellectual disability carry differing varieties of stigma, the impact of social attitudes can add pressure to a marriage.

This is what I understand when I read these studies: stress accretes, pressure builds, crises accumulate. Without support, even the strongest bonds strain. Mind-body difference in one person affects mind-body difference in another; we live in relation. Without support, the impact of disability ripples outward. I also understand that I didn't change fast enough to adapt to the changes in my life. I didn't alter my own ambition. I didn't relinquish the pressure on myself, and I didn't release pressure on Abel. I kept moving forward with plans—The Plan—instead of revising them. High. Functioning. Anxiety. Given all the pressure, it shouldn't have felt so surprising to see our marriage fracture beyond repair.

* * *

We returned from Ireland at the end of May, and I felt ready for a productive summer: I'd plant out my garden, head to Russia for two weeks with colleagues to scout out a study-abroad site, hang out at home for a couple more weeks, then head to a two-week writing residency in Nebraska at the end of July. I'd said yes to the Russia trip after the fourth miscarriage when escape to anywhere seemed like a good choice, and I'd applied for the residency unsure if I'd even be awarded it. When both worked out, Abel encouraged me to say yes to both.

I should've known how fragile these plans were, but they comforted me and propelled me forward as The Plan had before. Sensing fragility but not stopping, I stepped through that summer as I'd trod upon the limestone in the Burren—with care and hope despite the ground moving each time my foot met the earth. Cracks multiplied across the summer.

I pressed too hard when I expected Abel to dig a new part of the garden so I could plant it before I left for Russia. I knew he hated gardening, but I still asked—and after a few hours, he handed me the shovel with a dirt-streaked hand. "Christine, I love you, but ..." The first time he'd given a condition, an exception.

I pressed too hard expecting to fly away to Russia for two weeks without emotional fallout. With every item of clothing I packed, my anxiety grew, culminating in a full-fledged panic attack—an hour of sobbing followed by hours of unpacking and repacking. And still, even as I listed all my anxieties about leaving Holden, I countered myself with my litany of safety: my plans for babysitters and visits from my mother. I'd worked hard to make sure Holden would be safe and Abel would have help if he needed it.

I pressed too hard on the idea that space could help our strained relationship. After I presented Holden with a Russian *Kung Fu Panda* poster and a set of nesting dolls; after I told Abel stories about the Gorky Museum, taking shots of vodka with professors in their department's conference room, and the ornate subway stops in Moscow; after I'd unpacked my travel guide and mini Russian dictionary—Abel and I were sitting on the couch when he told me, "I'm not sure I want to be married anymore." I sat with that news, wondering what it meant exactly. Was he leaving me? He said he didn't want a divorce.

I pressed too hard on my coping mechanism: research. At the Kimmel Harding Nelson Center for the Arts in Nebraska City, a four-hour drive south down I-29 from Brookings, I woke up each morning and wrote with a mixture of guilt and relief. Guilt for leaving Holden again after being home from Russia only three weeks. Relief at escaping the stress of Abel's uncertainty and the silence between us that resulted. Sometimes, I fell into the writing, taking breaks for tea or to stretch my legs. Sometimes, I obsessed, reading internet articles such as "How to Save Your Marriage." Sometimes, I wrote love poems about us. Poems about our courtship focused my attention on what drew us together, and I hoped remembering all the joy we'd shared would keep us together. Writing to remember and to discover doubled here, my methods layering. I wanted my next book of poetry to celebrate love, and I planned to go home to a love to celebrate.

But evidence of fracture was everywhere when I returned after the residency ended. Abel avoided me at home, and he avoided me when we were out. He walked away from me when I tried to talk to him about anything—the writing I'd accomplished, what we needed at the grocery store. Finally, he told me: "I was happier this summer. Happier when you weren't home."

* * *

After Holden found the spiral shell in Ireland, I remember walking back to the car, worried that every step not only meant a crack in the thin shale but potentially crushing something lovely underneath. I wanted to move through the cracks in my life carefully. When Abel told me that he was happier when I wasn't home, part of me insisted on restraint. I'd wanted that kind of honesty. If he saw me hearing him openly and not losing my shit—if I gave him the space to work things out in his head—perhaps we'd arrive at the same place and fix our relationship.

The night my marriage ended, the afternoon had been so perfect that I believed our relationship was turning around. On the second Saturday in September, Abel, Holden, and I drove to an orchard in Sioux Falls to pick apples. The gravel in the parking lot crunched under our tires, and the sun felt warm. All three of us were smiling as we walked toward the apple stand. A clerk detailed the procedure and gave us buckets, pointing at a trolley.

"We get to ride *this* to pick apples?" Holden's eyes sparkled. Indeed. Once the trolley stopped, we scattered into the orchard with the other families. The air smelled of apples and cut hay—the end of summer.

"Let's pick those." Holden reached for a cluster of red apples in a tree high above him. In a few years, he'll be able to climb them, I thought. I recalled the nurse practitioner telling us to keep Holden away from heights. Worry flickered up, but I pushed it away. Abel hoisted Holden onto his shoulders, Holden's tan shorts against Abel's grey T-shirt. Holden's socks were pulled up to his knees, and already one was streaked with dirt.

I stepped back, right hand on my hip, and pushed my hair out of my eyes. Holden was such a blend of us. His hair curled at the end—both texture and colour a mix of his father's and mine. Holden had my face shape and lips, but his father's eyes and chin. But when the two reached for apples just above Holden's head, I saw how their mannerisms matched. They even dropped the apples into the bucket in the exact same way.

I followed Abel and Holden, practically skipping from tree to tree. The affection between them strengthened my optimism. The night before, Abel and I had attended a cooking class at our local grocery store, and we'd had a good time. We need more weekends like this, I thought. With Holden in kindergarten, we could settle into a schedule that would enable better planning. Time would make the epilepsy easier to manage. Abel and I could turn our relationship around.

"Pick this apple," Abel told Holden. "That one has a worm. See the hole?" Holden squealed, looking down at me. I gave him a thumbs-up. Abel and Holden grinned.

That evening, after dinner and a bath and a book, Abel tucked Holden in, and I took my seat at the counter. I opened my laptop to bookmarked websites about marriage problems and solutions. I'd searched for something concrete to propose to Abel. Almost every source mentioned spending more time together, reigniting common passions and interests, and being committed to open communication. We both loved martial arts and travel, reading and movies; Holden's epilepsy challenged some of these activities, but it didn't have to end them.

Abel walked around the corner from Holden's room, ready to head downstairs.

"Hey, wait," I said. "Let's talk about things." I smiled at him. He nodded and sat down next to me in his usual spot, yet at an angle so we faced each other. "I've been doing a bit of research on marriage, and I just think we need to work on our relationship with more intention. Today was really fun family time. We had a great date night last night, so it looks like we're already starting to do that." In that moment, I didn't realize that I was using all the good energy we'd shared that weekend to propel us forward. I didn't realize that I was analyzing what had just happened even as it was still happening or that we could've just left the weekend as we'd experienced it and put off our conversation to another day. "Improving our relationship will take a lot of work, but I think it's worth it."

I knew, even in that moment, that I was always looking for the key, the solution, the lesson. When Theresa died, I thought that if I could learn something from her life or make positive changes in my own, I could redeem her death. "Her death wouldn't be in vain," I'd said, as a dramatic preteen would. I knew, as I sat in the kitchen, that problems could be solved with work and creativity. Such were my core practices, the cornerstones of everything I'd built in my life. And I knew that I loved Abel, and I loved our family, and I wanted us to feel in love as we once were.

Silence cued me to look up from my laptop. Abel was looking at me.

"I've been thinking." His eyes held my gaze. "I don't think so." I stared at him and blinked. His posture was upright, and his voice was confident. Had I heard him correctly? "I don't want to work on it."

I shifted my focus. I drew breath through my nose, and I exhaled it out of my mouth. The room grew a bit fuzzy. *Inhale. Exhale. Inhale. Exhale.*

Then it clicked. Like a riddle solved. Like a lock picked. Like a puzzle piece placed to complete the image. This wasn't something he had *just* realized. He'd stopped working on our relationship long ago. Weeks? Months? The alignment of actions and words made everything clear and every vow undone.

I considered myself resilient. I kept an eye out for serendipity, for places to plant seeds to nurture happiness. I can't have another baby? We'll adopt. Don't want to adopt? We'll have adventures as a family of three. And that summer I tried to make that happen. Maybe this was a flaw. Maybe this masked or distorted reality. Maybe this made me a difficult person. Maybe the shattered pane of our marriage was all my fault.

"Even if I were to file tomorrow," Abel said, "the divorce wouldn't be final for two months." Divorce? How long had he known that he wanted a divorce? How long had he known that detail—how long a divorce takes in South Dakota? He'd been researching it. He'd been preparing. And I'd missed it. He continued, "I don't regret meeting you. I don't regret marrying you. I don't regret—"

"Stop! Don't say those things," I interrupted. Rage exploded in my chest and filled my lungs, my throat. It flickered behind my eyes. This wasn't a teenage breakup; it was a marriage. We had a child. This wasn't the time for a fucking speech.

"*If* you had regrets? *If*?" Was I yelling? I was yelling. I focused my voice until it sharpened into a needle: "If you had regrets"—I looked him in the eye—"I'd *hate* you." I snapped my laptop shut and walked into our bedroom, sobbing. I twisted my wedding ring off and buried it in my jewellery box. The words we exchanged and the ring put on married us; the words he said and the ring taken off divorced us.

Chapter Six

INTERMITTENT: stopping unpredictably

THREE WEEKS BEFORE THE DAY IN THE ORCHARD AND THE evening in the kitchen, I'd waited in the foyer of SDSU's "lab school" kindergarten with other parents eager to hear first-day stories. From the hallway lined with cubbies and coat hooks, I watched twenty-one kids mill about, a few I knew from Holden's preschool class. I hoped familiar faces had made his day easier; that morning he'd approached the classroom with nervous excitement.

Holden spotted me just as the teacher dismissed the class. "Mommy!" He ran to me, and we hugged. I brushed his hair with my hand, a curl sticking to his skin.

"How was your day?" I asked. He didn't answer. Instead, he pulled my arm toward the door. I wanted details—which kid said what silly thing, what he worried about, what games he played. "Holden, how was your day?" I asked again. Silence. He continued to pull on my arm. As I slipped his superhero backpack off the hook, his teacher, Mrs. Lewis, approached us.

"Do you have a minute?" she asked. Her voice had the quality of flannel, soft and strong. She waited until the other families filed out to continue. "Holden had a hard time following my directions today. When the class was sitting on the floor for instruction, for example, he'd want to get up and play with something or work at a table. I'd need to pause and redirect him, but it didn't happen just once. He kept needing to be redirected to stay on task the whole day."

"Oh." My earlier optimism faded. "Isn't that normal?"

"Yes, a bit, but not this extreme. He's very impulsive." Defensiveness flared up. I associated impulsivity with behaviour problems. Bad kids. Bad parenting. Mrs. Lewis switched gears. "I can tell Holden is sweet and intelligent, but if today was any indication, we'll have some trouble with him in the classroom this semester."

"It could be his epilepsy medication," I said. I'd emailed a handout on seizure first aid, but I hadn't mentioned the odd behaviour for fear of creating self-fulfilling expectations. "Did you notice anything else?"

"He seems very tired."

"His anti-seizure medication has a litany of side effects." I repeated my self-talk to her.

"I understand." Her voice lowered, and she turned from watching Holden run his fingers along the cubbies to look at me. "Christine, I'm going to need some help—besides my teaching assistant—if we want things to run smoothly this year." Was she implying that she didn't want Holden in her classroom? Did she think he was a bad kid? "I think we need to call in the district psychologist and get him evaluated," she continued. "That way, if a diagnosis comes back, we can use that to get additional help for him—maybe an aide."

His preschool teachers hadn't reported any problems. Had he changed so much over the summer? Was kindergarten that much harder?

I looked at Mrs. Lewis, and she held my gaze. She had kind eyes, and her face was non-judgmental. She wasn't stepping away from Holden; she was leaning in. She cared about the learning of her other twenty students, but she also cared about Holden.

"Okay," I said. I unfolded my arms and tucked some hair behind my ear. "I'll talk to his dad about it, and I'll call Dr. Porter, his neurologist, to seek her advice."

When I told a nurse in Dr. Porter's office what Mrs. Lewis had said, she explained impulsivity as a sign of ADHD—something often diagnosed alongside epilepsy. Our discussion resulted in a plan for Dr. Porter to write a letter in support of the school district's testing.

The Brookings School District acted quickly. Just after Labour Day, Abel and I received the Conners Test—Parent Form, a diagnostic tool for ADHD. After Holden fell asleep, we sat in our usual spots at the counter, bubble sheet and number-two pencil in front of me, questions in front of Abel.

"Does he have trouble with memory acquisition and management?" Abel asked.

"Yes. I ask him to grab his backpack from his bedroom, and I find him playing in the hallway, distracted by a toy." Abel nodded and I filled in the bubbles.

"Can he plan activities or complete tasks?"

"Rarely. He leaves puzzles half-finished. Although when he's interacting with one of us, he can focus for nearly fifteen minutes." I filled in the bubble for "Often."

When we'd finished the form, Holden met more than the requisite eight criteria for an ADHD diagnosis. This paperwork felt significant, as if we had agreed to say something about our son that carried weight.

"What happens if they say he has ADHD?" I asked. I imagined Holden's mind struggling to still, to focus on a blank sheet, an empty canvas, a pile of blocks. And holding still. Whereas my mind fell deep into the flow of the holding, perhaps a whiff of cookies or a flash of colour or a whisper from a kid sitting next to him yanked Holden away from concentration.

"I guess we'll see what the doctor suggests. What the teachers say," Abel replied, walking into the living room. He settled on the couch and picked up the remote. A week later, he'd say divorce.

* * *

Medical professionals categorize ADHD as a neurodevelopmental disorder affecting 11 percent of school-age children.[1] Resource websites, such as those published by CHADD (Children and Adults with Attention-Deficit/Hyperactivity Disorder) and similar groups, describe symptoms along the same lines: children with ADHD often squirm and fidget; they fail to finish tasks and act disorganized; they lose toys and forget chores; they talk or hum or sing. Impulsive, they interrupt and intrude. CHADD outlines information for children and their parents as well as adults with ADHD, publishing guides and outlining ways to find support. Despite these important resources, the website often uses language that frames ADHD within the medical model. For example, under the "For Parents" paragraph, it reads: "While ADHD is believed to be hereditary, effectively managing your child's symptoms can affect both the severity of the disorder and development of more serious problems over time.... The earlier you address your child's problems, the more likely you will be able to prevent school and social failure and associated problems such as under-achievement and poor self-esteem."[2] This wording locates the problem of ADHD in the child without considering that what disables children is that they must move through spaces, especially learning environments, not designed for them.

Functional imaging studies show the brains of children with ADHD are slightly different from the brains of children without ADHD.[3] For me, this suggestion of neurobiological difference frames ADHD as a natural human variation, and I want to appreciate the range and depth of natural human variation. I've observed that children with ADHD, however, are often treated as abnormal by learning institutions. What the children do or don't do draws attention. Their *behaviour* is scrutinized.

My first invitation to think about behaviour in children happened in my educational psychology courses as an undergraduate. I recall the emphasis on *training* students through positive reinforcement. If they raised their hand to speak, if they scored well on a quiz, and if they kept their work neat, I could reinforce these responses by allocating points, awarding higher grades, or drawing stars on the board beside their names. I could even distribute candy on special occasions. I related these techniques to Pavlov's dogs salivating when they heard a bell—classical conditioning. I thought about B.F. Skinner's boxes where rats could press on a bar to receive food. These theories seemed so practical compared to the other kinds of psychology I learned about in literature coursework—Freud and psychoanalysis explaining how our unconscious minds dictate our wishes, desires, and actions. I enjoyed analyzing a character's interplay of ego and id in a novel because speculating was so much fun, but it didn't help with the classroom management plans my education professors asked me to create.

Although I hadn't yet thought about these theories explicitly as frames, as lenses, I used them as such. Discounting psychoanalysis meant I didn't need to look inside the frame of internal thoughts. I didn't need to wonder about students' inner lives in order to understand what motivated them. My frame focused my energy on shaping their behaviour as I could *see* it. And I think that's how Mrs. Lewis saw it too.

Although she didn't use any labels to define Holden the day she pulled me aside, when I met the school district's psychologist a few weeks later, she shared Mrs. Lewis's ADHD assessment for Holden. I read the list, and I swallowed hard. Her observations indicated more than a lack of focus. They included not following directions, wandering away from class activities, and taking things without asking. She also noted that he would ask for things regarding physical needs, like hunger or thirst, but had not been observed asking questions like clarifications, questions regarding his schoolwork, or expressing his likes or dislikes. Holden often needed verbal reminders, and she had not observed him initiating social interactions with his peers.

Mrs. Lewis's assertions plopped into my mind like stones in a pond, crashing through the surface of understanding. I read the list twice, crossing my legs the second time and pulling my arms closer. I tried to counter her observations with my own. The list included Holden making fleeting eye contact, but he had made sustained eye contact with me—just that morning, actually. And he often told me what he liked and didn't like. Did Mrs. Lewis even know Holden? Maybe there wasn't anything wrong with him; maybe it was her. Maybe he wasn't adjusting to the school environment appropriately because it was faulty.

But the list pulled my attention back, and I read it again. This time, I exhaled at the end, trying not to let a few angry tears fly. Mrs. Lewis's words sank into my body and the ripples widened out; I knew they held some truth. I'd seen plenty of examples of everything on the list to know they weren't exaggerations. Just because Holden could negotiate personal space once or twice didn't mean it happened all the time. Even though he could tell me what he needed today didn't mean he did consistently.

I set the letter down and leaned forward, elbows on my knees, head in my hands. Holden used to be able to do all these things and more. He had made friends on a soccer field in Germany and had run around the children's museum with his friends Elif and Sam. How could his behaviour be in such flux? How could he do simple tasks sometimes but not always? How could all of these changes result from epilepsy?

When I posed these questions to the district psychologist, she brushed them aside. For her, ADHD was the answer, and she had a host of suggestions that could help me shape Holden's behaviour at home. I could place busy boxes—baskets filled with toys, colouring books, puzzles, and small sets of LEGO—around the house so there'd always be one within Holden's reach. I could reinforce Holden's good choices with rewards: video games, puzzles, costumes, board games. I could use a sticker chart, too, for more reinforcement.

With an ADHD diagnosis, Holden could receive his own Individualized Education Plan (IEP). From my undergraduate education courses, I knew teachers and parents designed IEPs to ensure that a child's particular learning needs were accommodated. For a child with a learning disability, for example, accommodations could include resources, therapies, or curriculum modifications. The IEP meeting seemed a good solution so Mrs. Lewis could have help in maintaining a classroom where Holden could learn and not disrupt his peers as he did so.

* * *

I don't remember much about the first few months after Abel said divorce, but my sense of self felt shredded. I walked around Brookings as if I had an open wound, blurting out the news to friends and acquaintances. I tried to stanch the bleeding with prolonged episodes of self-analysis:

What was wrong with me? What had I done wrong? Answers arrived cloaked in self-blame: you were too rigid, too perfectionistic; you were too focused on what you wanted, too driven. I scrutinized my own behaviour, cataloguing fights I'd picked and enumerating my odd, annoying habits. I conjectured that there might be other things, too—disappointing tendencies I didn't know about myself or didn't want to face.

I came close to believing that I wasn't worthy of love, and so I began to counter my perceptions. When self-blame popped up, I reminded myself of the things I'd done right: trying to work on the marriage, my willingness to change. Whenever I felt a prick of desperation, I repeated *You deserve to be loved by someone who wants to be with you* until I began to believe it emotionally and intellectually. By clinging to the self-confidence I'd built so deliberately in my twenties and holding tight to my feelings of self-worth, I resisted spiralling into self-hate. And when my self-talk failed to work, I called a friend or phoned my mom, and their pep talks gave me a boost.

Day to day, I tried to avoid Abel so I could manage my pain enough to do my job. When we had to interact, he was upbeat. There was a softness in his voice, a lilt sometimes. He acted as if a burden had been lifted. I was the burden. Yet his kindness hurt, even if it was better than apathy or anger. Divorce from me was all he needed for happiness, I thought.

Braided into the emotional mix was worry regarding my ability to parent Holden alone. The idea of solo parenting terrified me. Abel still lived in our house while we figured out logistics—paying down our debt so two households would be possible. But I imagined what it would be like once Abel left. If Holden needed a drink of water, help with homework, an appointment made, or a nightmare quelled, I must provide it. If Holden spit out his medicine, crushed it with his finger, or ran out completely, I must troubleshoot. If Holden got a cold, the flu, or strep throat, I must watch for seizures all night long. If Holden broke a window, ruined the carpet, or unplugged the refrigerator, I must fix it. If Holden couldn't sleep, I must stay up with him. If Holden had a seizure, I must give the emergency medication. At home, I would be the one to keep Holden healthy and alive. I'd have to do all of this while maintaining work responsibilities, too. Failure felt probable.

By January, a sense of clarity—that Abel's actions and words aligned—steadied me a bit. With the psychological suspension dissolved, I could reclaim some strength and focus. And when Mrs. Lewis scheduled an IEP meeting for Holden, I was glad to have the mental bandwidth to concentrate.

* * *

Most websites describe ADHD as a behaviour issue—not reflective of a child's intelligence. Like epilepsy, ADHD shouldn't affect Holden's cognition. Before the meeting, I'd imagined that Mrs. Lewis would make modifications so that he could learn better and that an assistant could help curb his impulsivity by keeping him engaged. When I interacted with him one-on-one at home, he seemed to stay on task better. I assumed that would be the assistant's job at school.

When Abel and I met with Holden's teacher and other school personnel one bitterly cold day in January, I assumed they'd called the IEP meeting so we could sign whatever paperwork they needed to hire an assistant. Quick and easy and friendly. But it only felt that way for the few minutes we discussed the weather.

Then the district psychologist passed a stack of papers to Abel and me across the conference table; it seemed that Mrs. Lewis and the special education resource teacher—both also present—had their copies before the meeting. The district psychologist explained how they'd administered an intelligence test designed for children and wanted to discuss Holden's results first. This confused me. I'd agreed to an IQ test because Mrs. Lewis explained it as a requirement of the process, so why did it need a discussion? From what I recalled about IQ from my educational psychology course, genetics bestowed a person with a range of intellectual potential, and education helped develop a mind toward achievement within that range; IQ stayed relatively stable throughout one's life. Wasn't Holden's intellectual foundation established? Wasn't this about ADHD?

I flipped through the report. When I found the results section, my eyes blurred a bit. Holden's scores were below where I thought they'd be. I felt a flicker of anger borne of cognitive dissonance.

My son used to be a curious, sharp kid hitting all his learning milestones, I thought. *In four months that changed. Why?* My confusion felt as impenetrable as the snowbanks outside.

"I've seen him accomplish these sorts of tasks at home—puzzles, problem-solving," I said when the district psychologist finished summarizing the test results. "And he's creative." I explained to them how three weeks before—just two weeks after he'd taken the intelligence test—Holden, my mother, and I went shopping in downtown Des Moines. I'd given Holden my camera for entertainment as we browsed. When I uploaded the photos he took, I was astonished by the number of balanced compositions. He'd caught interesting patterns, like a cow-print purse next to a wooden lamp. He'd captured the sparkle on costume jewellery, perfectly framed a wall of kitchen knives, and zoomed in on his grandmother's hand holding stainless-steel measuring cups. He'd taken photos of the butterfly tattoo on my foot, exposed just below the cuff of my jeans, and one of his grandmother window-shopping. My favourite was of Holden's reflection in a window, his hands holding the camera, a taped-up flyer obscuring the rest of his face.

"I've seen him accomplish creative tasks," said Mrs. Lewis. "Just not consistently."

"His abilities fluctuate," I said. "I just don't understand it." My voice trailed off. Abel echoed my experiences; he'd seen Holden accomplish all sorts of intellectual tasks too.

"What could account for this randomness?" I asked. No one answered. Their expressions revealed concern but not curiosity. No one made suggestions or voiced their worry out loud. It seemed they accepted the test results without any thought to why. What mattered, it seemed, was what they could observe about his behaviour.

Evidence started to coalesce that made me ask why. Dr. Porter's letter supporting Holden's ADHD diagnosis, dated November 1, described his epilepsy in boilerplate language and explained how a child could be sleepy after a seizure. Then she noted that "behaviour problems may arise from ADHD and depression associated with seizures"—another tangled mess of cause and effect. In her more specific description of Holden, she included a sentence I read and reread: "The area of the brain from which seizures arise may be non-functional, leading to learning disabilities." Every website I'd read argued that seizures didn't affect cognition. After the overnight EEG, Dr. Porter had said to watch for learning problems, which I interpreted to mean Holden might be too tired to focus some days. But Holden knew his letters and sounds last year, and he could count and do simple addition. Were these the learning problems she'd cautioned me about?

In the moment of the meeting, despite recalling what Dr. Porter had written and said, I didn't know what the IQ test proved about my son, if anything. Unsettled, I just wanted to go home.

The resource teacher slid documents over for us to sign, and we left with learning objectives and an IEP that specified Holden would receive one-on-one help to achieve them. The objectives seemed written for any kindergartener, so their existence confused me. What had just happened? I knew the paper-pushing obscured something, even if I couldn't name it. It seemed we'd gone into the meeting with Holden's ADHD as the focus and left with a new framework: Holden wasn't *smart*.

And it seemed the district psychologist had her own explanation for Holden's intelligence scores—naughtiness. That night I read her report notes and saw the lens from which she viewed Holden—a lens that had changed from just a few months before, when she'd diagnosed him with ADHD. She'd recorded the difficulty she experienced administering the test to him, describing how he "insisted on moving away from the stimulus items and turned his back to the examiner. He would stare at the stimulus materials and would not say or do anything." She wondered if it was an example of passive refusal.

The district psychologist blamed a five-year-old for trying to manipulate the situation in a somewhat sophisticated way, but he had no reason to do this. She implied that he misbehaved on purpose, which wasn't consistent with my understanding of my son. Why would he choose this kind of behaviour? Why would any child? I wondered how much Holden's ADHD shaped the administration of the intelligence test and how much his behaviour affected his scores. I wondered how epilepsy and medications influenced the testing, and I wondered why the district psychologist hadn't mentioned these possibilities in the meeting or in her report. She focused on his behaviour, assuming he was in control of himself.

Seeing my child through this new frame, especially with the dual focus on intelligence and behaviour, made him seem like a different kid. I couldn't reconcile this, nor could I reconcile the changes in Holden. If I couldn't explain them, and I couldn't seem to help him, was I failing as a mother? I began to think I was.

When I look back, I can see with more clarity how each framework I used to understand Holden focused my attention in one place while obscuring others. Perhaps that's what the professionals had done as well. Behaviour meant listening and compliance with directions. Educational psychology theory addressed reinforcing good behaviour with praise and sticker charts. ADHD meant curbing impulsivity and lack of focus with one-on-one engagement and busy boxes. Epilepsy meant a rigid medication schedule and safety vigilance. Each time I peered into one frame, the rest blurred. And that also precluded me from speculating on their connections. I couldn't hold all these realities in my head simultaneously.

Yet I did assign one point of meaning to the IQ test: Holden was changing in crucial ways. My desperation to help him wore me down. I reported the IEP meeting and test results to Dr. Porter, and she offered to prescribe something for ADHD even though most kids with this diagnosis didn't start medication for many more years. Because she didn't insist on a clinic visit, I described my concerns about stimulants like Adderall and Ritalin over the phone. Those drugs, in addition to his others, seemed particularly stressful on a kid's body. Medication websites also listed significant possible side effects, such as irregular heartbeat, delirium, panic, and psychosis. I'd also found information warning against dependency. Dr. Porter suggested the non-stimulant ADHD medication Intuniv, which sounded better than the other options. I surrendered my fears about adding another medication to Holden's cocktail of Depakote and Valium. Dr. Porter said it might take up to six weeks to see change.

* * *

That spring, amid episodes of apathy and meltdowns, Holden and I found moments of fun. At the children's museum, he scooped sand in the dinosaur bone pit, sat still to get his face painted, and tossed plastic balls into a whirlpool. We attended a school fundraiser carnival where he played PLINKO and took turns fishing for prizes with other kids. He used his prize tickets to buy a Berenstain Bears book and three-eyed alien toy. At home, he donned a lab coat, and we changed two vials of clear liquid into red and blue with white powder; then we turned those liquids into gels. In the photo I snapped of our project, he's holding a plate of beakers and pipettes with three plastic cups of gel in the centre. His smile beams pride.

That spring, I focused on my writing, too. I'd won a fellowship at the South Dakota Art Museum to write poems based on art—ekphrastic poems. In a windowless room with wall-to-wall bookshelves, I sifted through the museum's collection on a computer, and for four hours each week, I sat in a metal folding chair studying paintings, drawings, or collages individually. Sometimes I described the imagery. Sometimes I researched the subject. Sometimes a curator and I discussed her knowledge of a piece. As I tapped out my notes on my laptop, I often interpreted the imagery, concepts, or emotions the art elicited alongside the frames of my experience. A tree's roots pushing into flecks of soil became *red weeds bloom* and a poem about divorce. I observed the grooved brushstrokes in an oil painting, marvelling at how the painter captured the vibrancy and fragility of the gladiolus, and wrote a poem about miscarriage. In response to a mixed-media print titled *Aquaform*, I drafted: *How is it that I see the body in so many of these paintings? These are cells, orange worms, blue membranes, islands of white space;* after many drafts, the poem centred on epilepsy. As my ekphrastic practice deepened, I realized that an artwork often became a frame to hold me. Art occupied my conscious mind, allowing me to play with language and puzzle out possibilities while simultaneously compelling my concerns. Everything intermingled, and new poems were produced. After working with the materials of sound, image, symbol, and metaphor, deep breaths became easier to take.

By April, I knew the Intuniv had failed to improve Holden's impulsivity and attention. Holden phased out more and more often with what appeared to me to be long absence seizures. He always seemed tired, and Mrs. Lewis reported that he fell asleep in school at least twice a week. She also said that he'd ripped a girl's pants, hit other children, and broken toys.

I told Helen all of this at his clinic visit that month, and I mentioned the fluctuating nature of his behaviour. But that day, she didn't see symptoms that worried her. Holden complied with all her poking and prodding—ears, eyes, throat, reflexes, and muscle strength. He walked across the room and jumped on one foot. His success satisfied her, and she sent him to the toy basket while she asked me more questions, including questions about school. I shared Mrs. Lewis's reports, which included phrases like "inconsistent progress and regression." She described Holden's abilities as "in flux" and his behaviour as "depressed." But Helen dismissed these concerns. "Sometimes children need more structure and motivation when it comes to making good choices about behaviour," she said. "I'll share these concerns with Dr. Porter and see you again in six months."

On the drive home, I fumed. I resented her insinuation that I wasn't giving him structure, that I wasn't able to motivate my child to choose good behaviour. I'd read articles about behaviour and employed charts. I fed him a good, balanced diet. I kept him on a regular sleep schedule. I spent quality time interacting with him. I used research and best practices, and planned to do the best I could. Holden wasn't a bad kid hell-bent on creating chaos. This didn't seem like a simple "not choosing good behaviour."[4]

It seemed that no one could put the right frame around the multiple images—EEG data, seizures, teaching testimonies, home narratives, and educational testing—to explain what was happening. Holden was falling through Dr. Porter's and Helen's diagnostic frames, falling through the cracks of their knowledge, and they didn't seem too concerned.

Holden was changing, and if I didn't find a reason why, I wouldn't be able to help him learn and laugh and smile with the same frequency as he once had. I felt as if I was losing Holden, and I knew I needed different or better help to keep him from disappearing. The second I walked in the door from the clinic visit with Helen, I threw down my bag, slid off my jacket, and picked up my phone to schedule an appointment with Holden's family doctor. I needed her help to accomplish the next step—finding a new neurologist.

* * *

Elements of behaviourism, as John Watson and B.F. Skinner framed them, were groundbreaking. As educators and psychologists interpreted behaviourist principles and expanded the theories' applications in the decades that followed, behaviourism became so rooted—so foundational—that it began to shape our attitudes about learning and behaviour without our awareness. It became an invisible frame.

It didn't seem possible to the district psychologist, or to Helen, or to any educational or medical professional that Holden's actions might stem from causes that their behaviourist techniques couldn't address. Dr. Porter implied that a learning problem could be caused by the seizure disorder but never explained how or why, or offered anything other than medication as a solution. The professionals I encountered sometimes conflated learning and behaviour, and at other times made them appear distinct.

Now I understand that, had I used the framework of disability, I might have reframed these experiences with medical professionals and educators.[5] I might have apprehended the gaps—what was missing in my attempts to explain the relationships among IQ tests, inventories, medications, and observations. Now I see the mistake we made in overemphasizing behaviour theory as a solution to the issues that kept popping up. Those who insisted I could motivate Holden to behave were missing a crucial piece of the puzzle. As I would learn later from a different neurologist, Holden's learning, focus, and behaviour were tied directly to his seizures—the type of seizures and the rate at which he experienced them.

* * *

At the end of April, when a judge finalized the divorce and Abel moved out, I felt completely alone. Abel planned to stay in Brookings, and he asked for joint custody with me as custodial parent, which meant he'd see Holden every other evening during the week, with the weekends split in half. Yet even this equitable arrangement felt untenable.

The afternoon he left, the three of us sat on Holden's bed to read a children's book about divorce. Holden curled into Abel's arms as he opened the book. We'd discussed divorce with him before, but the conversations didn't seem to click. Abel's moving out, I imagined, would make it concrete.

Abel looked at me. I looked at him. I fought back the urge to wrap myself around them both one last time, and I fought the sadness settling in my chest.

"Why don't you read the book?" I asked. My voice sounded thin. Abel began to read about the main character now having two bedrooms, two homes, and two parents who loved him all the same but lived separately. As Holden turned the pages, I remembered that last big seizure Abel heard on the monitor. I remembered Abel's steady presence in emergency rooms and his trips to the pharmacy on cold nights when we'd run out of Holden's medication.

Although Abel promised to be close by and be there for Holden, all the cooking, cleaning, appointment-making, medication-wrangling, bill-paying, and budget-minding would be mine alone. Plus my professorship. My writing. A myriad of work-related responsibilities. *I'll need to keep doing a good job at work,* I thought. I was up for tenure the next year. I needed the income and health insurance for Holden. Each insight pushed more breath out of me until I coughed a bit.

"Are you okay?" Holden asked. "Daddy's reading this book to me!"

"I'm okay." I took a deep breath, and I felt my body shift toward Holden. Abel read the last page and closed the book.

"Holden, do you understand what the book said?" Abel asked.

"Yes!" he said, smiling. He was eager to hug his father, and he clung to him a few seconds longer than usual before Abel walked out the door.

So much about our lives was changing. No frame I could access helped explain any of it.

Chapter Seven

INTERNAL: situated on the inside

ONE LATE AFTERNOON IN JUNE, HOLDEN WANDERED THROUGH the house. In his bedroom, he turned over his action-figure bin, LEGO bin, block bin, and train bin one by one, toys flying through the air. Batman and Iron Man drowned in a mound of LEGO. Wooden cubes covered a plastic caboose. Holden stomped through the piles, kicking some toys, crushing others. His face was blank. He ducked under my arm, which held the door open.

In my bedroom, Holden opened my great-grandmother's candy tin, scooped up a handful of costume jewellery, and flung it. Pearls slid down the wall. He looked around as if searching for another projectile.

"Knock it off!" I said. His head dropped, and he pushed me out of the way.

He calmed down for a bit, so I started assembling dinner. Meanwhile, he pushed a stool to the pantry, grabbed a canister of sugar, and lugged it ten feet to the living room. When I turned around, he was dumping sugar onto the floor.

"What are you doing?" I asked. He blinked, as if my voice were a roll of thunder he couldn't quite place. "Clean this up now, or else you'll lose a magnet on your chart." I put down the carrot in my hand and took three steps to his behaviour chart on the wall. I pointed to one smiley-face magnet. Holden didn't move. I touched it with my fingertip; he still didn't move. He just kept looking at me. Jaw set, I started to pluck off the magnet.

"No!" he said.

"If you don't want to lose one, clean up that mess," I said.

"No!" he said. I removed the magnet. "No!" I removed another. He stood there, still.

"Time-out." I dragged the stool to the centre of the kitchen.

"Hmmph!" Holden said.

"Now." My voice was firm, calm.

"No!" He kicked the pile of sugar. Crystals flew through the air and landed on the couch, the television, the piano. Anger rippled through my body, and the muscles in my arms tensed. I picked him up. His body stiffened—arms at his sides, legs straight. I lugged him over to the chair, but I couldn't physically make him sit.

"Fine. Bedtime. Go to your room." I half picked up, half pushed him toward his door.

"No!" he screamed. "No! No!" He muttered a stream of garbled syllables. I heard the word *pajamas*. From his dresser, I fished out some blue shorts with white sharks and held them out. "Nuh-huh," he said, shaking his head. Perhaps he'd calm down with them on, I thought.

As I peeled off his T-shirt, he threw himself on his bed. My anger moved outward to the tips of my hands and feet. I waved the pajamas as if to say, *Here they are! Right here!* He pulled off his shorts and ran, naked, into the living room.

"Why not get your jammies on, Holden?" I followed him. "Isn't that what you wanted?" Why didn't he just tell me what he wanted? "You don't have to go to sleep now—just get ready."

"No!" he yelled again. He crept toward the front door. I stood between him and the door in case he decided to bolt. The hot sun, magnified by the door's window, warmed my back.

"Why are you doing this?" My voice was a harsh whisper. "Why don't you just get dressed?" Holden backed up against the coat closet.

"I want Dad!" he said. *He's punishing me for the divorce,* I thought. I loomed over him, hands on my hips, shaking with anger.

"It's not my fault your dad isn't here!" I yelled.

"Yes it *is*!" Holden screamed. He looked at me; I looked at him. We held each other's gazes. His directness shocked me. As I thought about how to interpret this—and how to respond—he urinated on the hardwood floor.

"Stop!" I screamed, stunned. The puddle grew. Desperation and anger twisted, intensifying. I recalled the day when Holden broke the glass—how he crawled up my back to get the shards, how nothing deterred him.

I grabbed his arm and turned him around and smacked his bare butt with my open palm. A red hand outline appeared.

He started to cry; I started to cry. He ran to my room, and I followed. He pulled the bedcovers up over his head.

"Why did you do that? Why did you pee on the floor?" I asked.

He didn't answer.

My time spent questioning my capacity as a parent and doubting my ability had increased over time, parallel with Holden's mysterious behaviour. But in that moment, crying on the bed with my son, I stopped wondering what I was doing wrong. The emotion moved beyond reason. Desperation sharpened and pierced something deep inside of me. I didn't feel unhinged or out of control; I felt absolutely hopeless. When I closed my eyes, I saw myself hovering over a gaping hole. I hoped sleep would welcome me into it.

Even though it was early evening, Holden and I both cried ourselves to sleep.

* * *

Andrew Solomon takes expansive dives into disability in his book *Far from the Tree: Parents, Children, and the Search for Identity*.[1] But first, he traces a theory from which readers can taxonomize kinds of identity. Vertical identities are those we inherit via our DNA or a family's cultural context: ethnicity, race, religion, language.[2] I learned, implicitly, what it meant to be white; I learned, explicitly at home, school, and church, what it meant to be Catholic. I learned to speak English with a midwestern accent, as did all the members of my family. And because I'm cisgender and straight, those identities were affirmed by my particular family. Had they not been, I could describe them as horizontal identities—traits inherent in or acquired by children that are different from their parents'. Horizontal identities, such as disability, autism, giftedness, and sexuality, are quite distinct from one another. What members of this group have in common is the need for peers for identity acquisition. Solomon writes that a gay child born to straight parents must learn "gay identity by observing and participating in a subculture outside the family," as he did.[3]

When I read Solomon's words eight years after the sugar-flinging episode, I thought through his theory by applying the transmission of identity to my life. I recalled how I had researched the possibility of adopting a child of a different race; I reflected on how I might react if my child came out as queer. Of course, I imagined loving across these differences, but I understood that only experience would reveal how that love would manifest. What garnered more insight was the absence of disability from my thoughts about parenting. With the exception of considering disability in relationship to chromosomal abnormality as a cause for miscarriage, I didn't remember seriously engaging the question, *What if my child is disabled?*

Solomon notes that the disjuncture between a parent's and child's identities can cause parents to misapprehend their children. When unexpected difference disrupts families, parents often respond by trying to change the child. Solomon writes, "Anomalous bodies are usually more frightening to people who witness them than to people who have them.... Labeling a child's mind as diseased—whether with autism, intellectual disabilities, or transgenderism—may reflect the discomfort that mind gives parents more than any discomfort it causes their child."[4]

I understood that discomfort, that fear. To the sugar-flinging and peeing incident, I added new words to my interpretation of *not normal*: wild, crazy, wrong. A scene from Helen Keller's biography, one I had read as a child, kept returning to me. Young Helen roamed her family's dining room, snatching sausages from everyone's plates. I remembered that character as out of control, as wild, as crazy, as wrong—especially since my father's strictness at mealtimes meant we often ate in silence and focused on the correct use of our silverware. The shock of Helen's behaviour seared the scene into my memory.[5] At times, Holden seemed similarly out of control.

I feel shame admitting that now. I wish I'd understood Helen Keller's behaviour as rational; without access to other forms of communication, Keller satisfied her needs any way she could. Likening Holden's behaviour to Helen's (assumed) irrationality pointed to my shallow interpretation of Holden as well. It would be a few months before I'd learn that his behaviour was not of his own making—not his choice. My ignorance points to my lack of knowledge regarding what was happening to Holden. Ideas of normalcy, behaviourist assumptions, and framing epilepsy strictly as a medical condition only heightened my fear.

* * *

The day after Holden and I cried ourselves to sleep, I drove ninety miles west along Highway 14 from Brookings to Huron for a poetry society board meeting. The night before haunted me as I sped along. Holden's outburst had made me afraid, but I was equally fearful of my reaction—I hadn't spanked him before. It stunned him, and he didn't seem to understand it. *I won't do that again,* I thought. Cornfield after cornfield, I replayed the scene, imagining different decisions: I could've walked away. I could've hugged him. I could've carried him to his room and shut the door. I could've dropped my voice and not yelled. Regardless of the permutations, I still felt desperate. The desperation unsettled me. My physical body felt lighter in weight, translucent in appearance. Looser. Off balance. I felt shorter and smaller, as though I could more easily disappear.

When a historical marker alongside the highway distracted me from my self-analysis, I decided to pull over and take a quick break. The marker described Manchester, a town incorporated in 1881 and destroyed by a F4 tornado 122 years later. With blue sky for miles, a puff of white cloud here and there, and tall green grass that touched the horizon, I couldn't imagine such a storm. When the tornado hit on June 24, 2003, the town contained fewer than a dozen buildings; luckily, most of its hundred residents farmed outside town limits. *That was less than ten years ago,* I thought. I looked to my left, imagining how the tornado widened into a wedge about the width of a mile as it entered the town from the south, its 260-mph winds sending wood and glass flying; concrete walls crumbled. A flag and the outline of a building commemorated Manchester's history. The water pump, directly hit by the tornado, remained. Nothing else did.

As I stood near that water pump under a calm sky, I realized that being Holden's mom felt like that day, that weather, that place; it was beautiful and peaceful and, at any moment, warm air could meet cold air the way the neurons in Holden's brain synched, a seizure or tantrum reducing everything to rubble.

But when a storm in the brain brought everything down, I didn't want to be scooped up by winds and thrown into the debris, broken. In those ten months since Abel said the word *divorce*, I'd had moments when I wanted to disappear whole. Like Dorothy in *The Wizard of Oz*, a tornado depositing her into a land of Technicolour and song, I wanted to disappear from my Kansas and spiral up and up and up into a place far, far away. Or maybe disappear into the earth, my body growing lighter until my flesh and bones merged with soil. Either way, I'd be gone, and I wouldn't hurt anymore.

If I closed my eyes and eclipsed the sun and the expanse of farmland, I could still see the gaping hole from the night before—a permanent precipice. When desperate, I told myself that my life didn't seem to have much impact. I wasn't able to influence Holden's behaviour or unpuzzle the tantrums. I wasn't able to inspire his father to stay in our marriage. I wasn't able to bring life forward again. I peered down that hole, and I felt the emptiness beckoning.

Although I've heard of families where multiple people have died young and unexpectedly, I couldn't contemplate my family as one. I couldn't bear the thought of adding any more sorrow to my parents' grief. I didn't want to hurt myself; I just wanted to stop hurting. I didn't want to die; I just wanted to be erased.[6]

I wanted erasure to sneak up on me as it had on Theresa—while I slept, numb to its approach. No one would know I'd thought about it, then. No one would know because I appeared in control, appeared to be doing well under the pressure of divorce, miscarriages, and a kid with epilepsy.

But I wasn't in control. The Plan had dissolved, or it had been an illusion all along. When desperate, I believed no other human being in history had felt as isolated as I did; at the same time, I felt that anyone could step into my life and manage my responsibilities just fine.

A breeze stirred the grass near the marker. A tornado had erased Manchester from the prairie. *Who carries the memories?* I wondered. Who stops here? I couldn't answer. "Keep your memories," I whispered to myself. "Keep moving. Either you'll disappear or you won't." Shaking, I slid back into my car.

* * *

In *Far from the Tree*, Solomon engages in deep conversations with families where horizontal identities challenged family dynamics. He wants us to understand how these families changed in order to shed light on the ways "intimacy with difference fosters its accommodation."[7] He argues that having "exceptional children exaggerates parental tendencies; those who would be bad parents become awful parents, but those who would be good parents often become extraordinary."[8]

After the Easter seizure episode—when I'd sat in the field rocking Holden and realized that I'd left the emergency seizure medication at home—any illusion that I could aspire to exceptional parenting vanished. An exceptional parent would always be prepared, be knowledgeable, be focused. She would be selfless and assertive, patient and strong. My aspirations of perfection dissipated as The Plan dissolved. Until the sugar flinging and peeing episode, I thought I could be decent—I could strive even if I failed. But that had changed. Self-doubt replaced my confidence.

I often wonder what would have happened if stress had released me into depression. I wonder what would have happened if my panic attacks had increased in frequency. How would my own mental illness have complicated my ability to adapt as Holden shifted, as his needs deepened, as my role as parent expanded and intensified? I wonder what would have happened to me—and to Holden—if I'd disappeared.

I see possible answers in the anecdotes written by other parents on the discussion boards I follow. In the dozens of posts by parents of disabled children, I see testimonies of stress: lack of financial resources, unresponsive school districts, dearth of family support, marital discord. When a parent queries about ways to cope, dozens respond with mental-health advice—therapy, medication, self-care. Desperation surfaces for some—perhaps most—of these parents at least once. Caregivers need assistance from communities, schools, and institutions to help us move from being good parents to being the kind of exceptional parents that Solomon describes.

* * *

One afternoon that summer, I watched Holden's words disappear in what felt like real time. We were grocery shopping with our cart semi-full when Holden announced that he needed the restroom. We detoured down a hall that ended with two washroom doors, a drinking fountain, and a bench.

"There's the men's room," I said, taking a seat.

Holden sat down next to me.

"Do you have to potty?" His face neither affirmed nor countered my question.

"It's right there." I pointed to the door.

He blinked.

Because he'd been acting so strangely, I took out my phone to record him, hoping to capture evidence of a seizure or odd behaviour. I swept the camera to the men's room sign and back to Holden. He stretched out his legs and swung them over the side of the bench, his back pushing into me.

"So, you don't want to go potty?"

Silence.

"Holden, will you answer me, please?"

"Taco shop," he said.

"We're not at the taco shop. We're at the grocery store. Do you have to go—"

"TA-CO SHOP." Holden enunciated the syllables. "Taco shop."

"Do you have to go?" I asked.

"Taco shop." This time his voice was just above a whisper. His face looked angelic, and his *Toy Story* T-shirt underscored his sweetness.

"Why aren't you answering my question?" I asked.

"Ta-co-shop." Holden slowed each syllable, as if it were the sound I didn't understand.

"What does that mean?"

"Taco shop."

"But what does that mean, 'taco shop'?"

"Ummm. It means. Um. Uhhh. I ... umm ... need ... to ... go ... to ... the ... men's ... room."

"Okay. Then why don't you go to the men's room?" My voice was crisp. "We're right across from it. It's right there."

"Ouch." Holden tried to climb onto the cart. He was quiet then, grasping for the cart. What was he thinking? I wondered. Did the cart distract him?

"Honey, why don't you go?" My voice softened.

"Cart." He started to push the cart.

"Do you have to go to the bathroom? Yes or no?"

He turned back around and put his face in my phone. "Cheese!"

"Yes, I know, I'm recording," I replied. "But I'm just asking you if you have to go." Holden stood up but didn't walk over to the door. "Okay, then. I'm just going to start shopping."

Holden took the cart, and I stopped the recording. The rest of our shopping trip was uneventful, and he didn't use the toilet until we got home. But I couldn't stop thinking about that exchange. The repetition. The confusion. With every example that pointed to worsening symptoms, I observed, noted, and waited; at the end of August, our appointment at the University of Minnesota would yield answers.

In April, I'd visited with Holden's family doctor regarding a second opinion. As she listened to my concerns, she observed Holden. He sat on the examining table and stared over my shoulder at the door, but he didn't seem to be seeing it. He wasn't curious about the blood-pressure cuff or the row of instruments within arm's reach. His brown eyes were dull, the bags beneath them more pronounced than usual. Later, this doctor would describe Holden at that visit as a zombie. "It was like no one was there," she'd say. During that appointment, she persuaded me that the University of Minnesota Hospital—a four-hour drive east from our home—would be the best place for a second opinion, and she promised to write a referral that day. Despite her quick action, the earliest appointment I could get was three months later, at the end of August.

* * *

While I waited for that appointment, I tried to find answers on my own. Dr. Porter had said that Holden's EEG pointed to an epilepsy syndrome, but it didn't fit the criteria exactly. Perhaps she was wrong. I researched epilepsy syndromes in earnest.

On the Epilepsy Foundation's website, epilepsy syndromes were defined as a cluster of features, including seizure type, age of seizure onset, seizure causes, genetic components, factors that provoke seizures, severity/patterns/frequency of seizures, EEG patterns, and prospects for recovery or worsening.[9] As I read about each syndrome, I deleted from my mental list those that clearly didn't fit Holden: Angelman syndrome was diagnosed in babies because of developmental delay, and seizures in benign rolandic epilepsy involved twitches. Childhood absence epilepsy was similar to the kind Helen had described, but didn't match up either. Seizures triggered by fever were linked to Doose syndrome, and because Holden's didn't always seem to be, I removed that one from the list. And so on.

Of the two dozen I read about, two made me pause: Continuous Spike and Wave during Sleep (CSWS) and Landau-Kleffner syndrome (LKS). I thought that CSWS could be a possibility because Dr. Porter had described the seizures on the overnight EEG as of the "slow wave and spike variety." The website associated CSWS with simple partial seizures, cluster seizures (a series of back-to-back seizures), and the need to treat clusters with emergency seizure medication. But Holden didn't have clusters, and Dr. Porter had described his bigger seizures as complex partial. (Simple partial and complex partial—now outdated terms—refer to how much of the brain is affected and whether consciousness is lost.) Plus, children with CSWS experienced "global cognitive regression." *How could cognitive capacities regress without some kind of brain injury or head trauma?* I wondered. *I wasn't seeing extreme cognitive problems with Holden, was I?*

As an undergraduate, I'd taken a course called Mainstreaming the Exceptional Child, which required service-learning work with disabled children. I shadowed a friend who worked in a group home near my house. For five hours, I cuddled a nine-year-old girl who couldn't speak. Sitting next to her on the sofa as the lives of her housemates swirled around us, I stroked her hair and pondered what it meant that her parents had moved to Texas and left her in Iowa. She'd been born healthy and developed normally; then, at some point, she regressed. Eventually, her systems would shut down and she would die. I knew cognitive regression as a sweet nine-year-old girl who needed attention so much that she curled up next to a stranger. When I juxtaposed Holden and the memory of her, there was no comparison. Clearly, I wasn't seeing signs of regression, I thought. I crossed CSWS off the list.

Holden fit many of the characteristics of LKS—age of seizure onset, seizure types, attention problems. But the hallmark symptom, "loss of language," didn't fit as perfectly as the rest. Was Holden losing language? He could still talk, I thought. He wasn't mute. But then, what did losing language look like? For me, loss meant all or nothing. I'd lost Theresa. I'd lost four pregnancies. If language was lost, it was gone, I reasoned. On other websites with LKS information, descriptions quickly went from basic to expert. The abstracts of medical articles my search turned up seemed to be written in another language entirely. When I saw the word *mutism* on the symptom list in one article, I grasped it. He wasn't mute, I thought. Because Holden could still speak, I scratched LKS off the possibilities list.

Now I realize that my lack of language to understand what I was observing affected my ignorance. I didn't comprehend disability; I could only see diagnosis. As I searched for diagnosis, I sought clear-cut distinctions, since my medically framed thinking trusted in a decisive, algorithmic approach to a solution: a combination of symptoms led to a few tests and then a prescription. I didn't yet know that I needed a new language. Solomon addresses this need for language in a slightly different way. "We often use *illness* to disparage a way of being, and *identity* to validate the same way of being. This is a false dichotomy.... Many conditions are both illness and identity, but we can see one only when we obscure the other. Identity politics refutes the idea of illness, while medicine shortchanges identity. Both are diminished by this narrowness."[10] It would be linking epilepsy and disability as Solomon suggests, as "compatible aspects of a condition," that would lead me to a more profound, complex, and useful way to interpret my role as Holden's mother. But that summer Holden was six years old, and my new understanding was still years away.[11]

If I'm totally honest with myself, there's a deeper fear that reading words like *regression* sparked in those moments of research. I'm ashamed I let that fear arrest my inquiry, but I'm fairly certain it did. I was in middle school when my mother told me that our cousins, Scott and Stacy—the children of her first cousin, Larry—had a fatal genetic condition. Their neurodegenerative disease caused their development to reverse at puberty. Much like the child I met at the group home, they lost their cognitive and physical abilities until they died. Both were twenty years and eight months old when they passed away.

Scott was six years older than me and Stacy three, and they lived on the opposite side of town from my family. Aside from occasional reunions, we didn't see my mom's cousins often. I remember bits and pieces: the fundraiser we attended to help support their family; their mother—a petite woman—lifting her teenaged son out of the car and into a wheelchair; Scott's and Stacy's burials—their graves in the same cemetery as Theresa's but in a different section. My mother held deep respect for their parents, especially their mother, Pam, who cared for them every day knowing she couldn't prevent their deaths.

Perhaps because Scott died just three years after Theresa, and Stacy three years after Scott, I buried that fear deep down with my own grief. I couldn't contemplate that kind of pain. I wonder, had I known then what I know now—that the cause of their deaths was an ultra-rare genetic kind of seizure disorder, Baltic Myoclonic Epilepsy—whether that knowledge would have changed my decisions as I advocated to find the right medical support for Holden.

* * *

In *Far from the Tree*, Solomon uses the dual nature of light (is light a particle or a wave?) to help make the argument that some conditions can be the result of both identity and illness. It depends on the perspective from which one looks, the nature of the questions one asks.[12] I feel that tension of two vantage points when I look back at that summer of taco-shop muttering.

Anxiety and fear unhinged me; I wanted to disappear.

And yet, when a thread of hope appeared, I grasped it.

That thread of hope? Love.

Chapter Eight

INTERCOURSE: exchange, communion, connection

"DIVORCE IS TOUGH, NO MATTER HOW AMICABLE IT MIGHT be," Brian said, stirring his latte. He leaned in. "It's been two years for me, and yet it seems like a whole different life."

Another SDSU colleague at our table shared an anecdote about his own breakup, but I just nodded along. It was late April, and my divorce from Abel had only been final for a week. I understood how the break could feel as profound as Brian described, but I couldn't imagine that for myself. Perhaps because of Holden. Perhaps because it was too new. Perhaps because I was no longer sliding along The Plan—that socially sanctioned, family-approved order—and I couldn't recognize my context. I felt like every person in the Cottonwood Café knew that, too. The English Club students who'd gathered for the open mic, the baristas who'd memorized my order history, the community members who recognized me as a regular—all of them either judging me or pitying me or both. Perhaps those worries were why I'd taken such care with my appearance that night: magenta sleeveless blouse, fitted jeans, sparkly necklace—all new. I needed to support my students, and I wanted to look presentable and happy and like I had my shit together even if I didn't, even if my heart ached with self-doubt.

When the conversation paused, everyone at our table took a sip. I wondered why my colleague insisted that I join him at his table with Brian. Perhaps he just didn't want to be stuck with the divorcée by himself. I'd been introduced to Brian at a meeting nearly two years prior when he was the brand-new leader of the architecture department; later, I fielded some questions he had about William Carlos Williams—an email that found me via a circuitous route of "Who can answer this guy's question?" I wasn't sure he recalled those previous encounters with me.

"Do you have any children, Brian?" I asked.

"Yes. A daughter. She lives with her mom in Canada, but she's coming to visit me this summer." A smile crossed his face; it was clear he missed her.

"That's something to look forward to. I have one child, too. A son. Holden. He's six." We chatted a few more minutes before the English Club's officers interrupted. Worried that not enough people had signed up for the open mic, they asked me to read a few poems. I agreed.

The program began with students reading pieces of short fiction. As I listened, I glanced over at Brian to see how he reacted to the work. He pushed his hair away from his black-framed glasses and took a sip of his coffee at the conclusion of every reader—an endearing pattern. Then a student called my name.

I felt myself step into the role of writer–professor as I stood. It'd taken me years to transition into that stance so quickly—a version of myself, a performance: organized, poised, passionate. All those years of reading, studying, and writing made it easier to actualize when I entered any kind of teaching space. I took a deep breath, stepped before the microphone, and felt the self-consciousness drop away.

"Thanks for asking me to read tonight," I said. "I don't have any of my books with me, but I do have some new poems here on my laptop." Balancing my computer on my arm, I looked around the room. A group of former students, a handful of current students, and some I didn't know sat among a few folks from Brookings who hadn't planned to crash an open mic. My eyes met Brian's. I slipped my hair behind my ear, and I smiled. For a second, I wondered if anyone guessed that I was smiling at him. "I'll read three. The first, 'All My Engineering,' I'll read for my new friend, the professor of architecture, since there's some architecture imagery in here somewhere ...

> I want to engineer
> us, so I sketch black lines
> on a future's blueprint, form
> squares with my fingers, press
> words into an art-deco-cubist-
> Frank-Lloyd-Wright something...."

As I read, I thought it odd that I'd written a poem with that reference, especially since I didn't know much about architecture. I wondered how Brian reacted to what I'd said, but my reading was too long for me to gauge. By the time I looked up, he was just looking at me, grinning.

* * *

In writing, a *palimpsest* results when someone erases words from a piece of material and the material is reused for new words. Traces of the earlier writing remain visible. Months later, when Brian taught me the architectural version of palimpsest—something altered but retaining visible traces of its former form—it became the perfect metaphor for what he and I had begun to do: trace a new relationship on the outlines of older ones. Bernard Tschumi theorizes that when confronted with an opportunity to build in an urban environment, an architect can analyze the historical layers and work upon those—a palimpsest.[1] In the beginning, Brian and I deconstructed our pasts by narrating the shapes of our lives that preceded our meeting. We exchanged emails chock full of images and stories, adding layers to the outlines of our lives before we met. Before we could even detail the uses of our space, Brian and I wrote on the traces and designed something new.

A few weeks after the poetry reading, I opened my laptop to find an email from Brian with the subject line "Paterson, Cottonwood, and

Things." *Seems he noticed my flirtation,* I thought. He'd remembered our conversation about William Carlos Williams and that I'd written that the poet-doctor's work "makes me swoon." Brian marvelled at the fact that poetry can "build a swoon," then confessed: "I know this for myself now. I think your kindness and beauty in words at that Cottonwood reading a few weeks ago gave me a bit of a swoon. I revel in the little fact that you read a piece for me. That was the perfect moment for someone to give me a creative notice. Thank you. I'd really like to get to know you better."

Shit! I thought, slamming my laptop shut. *What do I do now?* I felt like a kid getting caught shoplifting candy. He wasn't supposed to notice, and he wasn't supposed to like me back. I felt seen, and I felt panicky. Since splitting with Abel, I'd accepted a few "date-like" invitations for lunches or coffees or drinks—diversions from the sadness of life after divorce. I enjoyed being around men who wanted to spend time with me, but second dates were rare. And that suited me fine because no one had sparked my interest the way Brian did. I reread his email throughout the day. *He's a good writer, and he'd taken a risk writing that email, too,* I thought. By late afternoon, I'd convinced myself that I needed to reply, but nerves paralyzed me. Finally, I pecked out a stilted "I'll compose a response to your email when I compose myself. I'd like to get to know you better, too."

I waited nearly two weeks to email again, though. Every time I thought about it, I worried. What if it became a relationship? Did I have the energy for one? What would people say about me starting something so soon after my divorce? With no answers, I stalled. But I kept thinking about him and about his lovely email and about how he brushed his thick hair away from his glasses. I decided to take a chance. *Just do something that makes you happy,* I thought. *It's only an email.*

My reply to Brian described the summer course I was preparing to teach and my struggle to adjust to my new life as a solo parent, but I also acknowledged that I'd been energized by our conversation. He wrote back in the style that typified his correspondence that summer—lyrical and story-filled: "I know exactly what you mean by overwhelmed. There is a middle ground of thoughts that fresh memories won't let me take up and work through. I am reading voraciously and really pushing myself to rethink 'what I profess.'" The gravity and passion with which he spoke about his work—he'd been a professor of architecture for nearly fifteen years—and the way he described his emotional process impressed me: "Scratching out a disciplinary stance in this university is making me see myself very naked. Divorce can be old hat one day and then crawling inside my clothes the next. It makes the lost marriage feel like itchy underwear." Brian's first marriage—started when he was just nineteen—lasted twenty-five years. I imagined how tough it would be to deconstruct that life and build anew.

An intense intellectual get-to-know-you fuelled our month-long email correspondence. Each weekday I'd wake up to an email—usually written at midnight or two in the morning—packed with stories and explorations of art and architecture.[2] He wrote with Texas-isms, mixed metaphors, and ample rhythm—all of which charmed me and built a connection between us. On June 10, I woke up to a description of the forty boxes of books he'd opened that day—forty of 200 boxes of architecture books he purchased from a historian in Portland, Oregon, for SDSU's library: "I make librarians blush with my love of books. I gush. They gush at the gush." Sitting alone in my kitchen, I'd imagined him lifting out one book at a time, cracking the spines, inhaling dust. I'd blushed, too, but waited until Holden was up and off to daycare before replying with a book story of my own.

Some emails analyzed our educational and professional paths, describing the indirect routes that led us to South Dakota and contrasting them with each other's. Between grading my online summer class and writing, I'd read about Brian's stint as a non-traditional student at a community college in Texas and how he eventually finished his education at Columbia in New York; once a draftsman, he was now building an architecture program. The feeling of *How did I get here?* was familiar to me. I wrote back: "I'm from a working-class family, too, and I'm one of the few university graduates in my extended family. If someone had told me, when I was sixteen, that I'd publish books and have a Ph.D., I would've said, 'Cool about the books, but what's a Ph.D.?'" His terminal degree was a master's in architecture, so in his response he teased me about outranking him.

Brian's emails waxed poetic, sometimes whimsical: "These last two years have been intellectually chaste—time breaking sod and living in a mud cave on the intellectual riverbank. Fresh water but no people." He charmed me. I didn't realize my hunger for intellectual intimacy until I read those words. His email continued: "Now, I'm sowing in earnest. You saw me try to come up out of the cave back with my missives about thing theory and W.C. Williams." I laughed out loud at how he mixed metaphor. He'd ask me questions, and throughout my day, as I cooked a meal or drove Holden to the park, I'd think about clever or interesting ways to respond. I never wrote lengthy letters back, but he kept writing pages and pages anyway. His attention meant that someone bright and engaged and creative—and cute—was interested. Interested in me.

* * *

Our email correspondence grew intense, and we both began to want to actually see each other. But teaching and parenting made that feel impossible. Just when Brian and I had discussed a date for dinner, Holden flung the sugar in the living room. Then, that day in Manchester when I contemplated tornadoes and disappearing, the emptiness beckoned its strongest. I wasn't sure I was ready for a date, never mind a relationship.

Our first date almost didn't happen because an incident with Holden caused me to melt down. I'd scheduled haircuts for both of us, then planned to meet Brian for dinner while Holden spent time with his dad.

"Holden, you're such a handsome guy!" Gigi said as we walked in the salon door. "Why don't you hop up here?" She pointed to a booster chair. Holden complied. She'd known us for several years, and Holden loved attention from Gigi.

"Cut the usual amount?" Gigi asked. I nodded. Holden shifted in his chair. I opened *Short Cuts* magazine and glanced through it. Holden squirmed when Gigi sprayed his hair with water, although none of it landed on his face. "Don't worry. It's just water," she said. With the jewellery-throwing episode vivid in my mind, I shifted into alert mode. When Holden tried to slip out of the chair, I sprung up and stood in front of him.

"C'mon, Holden." I scooted him back. "You know the drill." Gigi put down the spray bottle and turned on the clippers. Holden didn't usually get super-short cuts—who would dismantle those adorable curls?—but short enough to stay out of his eyes. As Gigi trimmed around his ears, Holden scrunched his shoulder to his ear and grimaced.

"You've had the clippers before," I said. "They don't hurt."

"Nope," said Gigi. "See?" She showed him how they tickled against her hand. His eyes lit up. She brought the clippers to his neck again.

"NO!" He pushed her arm away. Gigi and I looked at each other. She turned her head to the side, as if asking a question.

"Should we try scissors?" she asked. I nodded. She clipped the top and front, but every time her hands moved close to his ears, Holden tried to leap from the chair.

"I'm done," he said. But Gigi wasn't quite done. As I moved to a different angle to see what was left—not much; we could have gotten by—I noticed the only other customer in the salon staring at me. When I met her gaze, she didn't look away. My face flushed.

Gigi quickly finished Holden's cut and motioned me back to the sink area to get my hair washed. Holden jumped in the chair next to me and we both extended our necks into the sinks. I glanced over and noticed Holden still had his Band-Aid on from a blood draw earlier in the day to check his Depakote level. He hated blood draws, but he didn't seem grouchy anymore, laughing as he pretended to wash his hair. I took a deep breath, releasing my stress a bit. Gigi was rinsing my sudsy scalp when Holden jumped up and disappeared around the corner.

"Can you check on him?" I asked. Gigi walked over to where she could see him.

"He's looking at the display of shampoos and conditioners," she said. *Shit*, I thought, wondering what he'd do next.

"We'd better hurry up, then," I said. The other hairstylist said something to Holden as Gigi towel-dried my hair. When I moved back to the front of the salon, black cape billowing behind me, Holden was taking the shampoo bottles off the shelf and setting them on the floor. He turned to me with a blank expression on his face, then smiled. "Put them back," I said. The conversation between the other stylist and the staring customer stopped. I knelt down on the floor to help him. He turned away.

"Remember the box of toys?" Gigi asked. She walked over to a chair in the lobby and pulled out a box from underneath it. Holden smiled. As he examined the action figures, I settled into Gigi's chair. "Just trimmed up, please," I said. "And dried if there's time."

As Gigi cut my hair, Holden made his way to the bottom of the box. The mirror revealed the other customer still staring at me. I closed my eyes. Snip, snip, snip. *Relax,* I thought. A drop of sweat slid down my back and absorbed into my waistband. I wouldn't have time to go home and change because Holden was scheduled to be with Abel from 4:30 to 7:30, and he was picking him up at the salon. Brian expected me at the restaurant at 4:45.

When I opened my eyes, the staring lady was looking toward the lobby door. I turned to see Holden standing in front of the nail polish display. He held a bottle, and he was untwisting the cap.

"Holden!" I yelled. "Stop!" He didn't look up. What was he going to do with the nail polish? I didn't paint my nails. Had he watched anyone paint nails? Would he try? I stepped out of the chair, my arm already reaching. I tugged the cape off with one hand, the other grasping as Holden turned the jar upside down, orange paint pooling onto the floor.[3]

Gigi was all poise and grace. She looked down at the paint and walked behind the counter as I held Holden back from stepping into the mess and making it worse. "What do I owe you, including the nail polish?" I gave her my credit card. With everyone's eyes on me, I situated myself between Holden and the door, almost pinning him against it. Holden stood quiet and still behind me. She rang the charge.

"I'm so sorry," I said.

"Don't worry about it. Really." She handed my card back to me. Holden and I walked out. I wondered how she would clean the mess up and whether the other ladies would discuss what they'd seen.

Abel met us in the parking lot, and after he and Holden left, I sat in my car inhaling the humid air. Heat seeped through my skin and sweat dampened my armpits. Moisture lined the back of my neck. When I exhaled, tears came with the choked-back breath. *Another parenting failure,* I thought. I didn't stop crying until the bottom of my shirt was wet with wiped-away tears and I remembered my date. It was 4:44.

"I can't go," I said out loud. I felt like crawling in bed and crying some more and dissolving the rest of the way. I took out my phone, found Brian's number, stared at the call icon, and rehearsed several times: "Hey, Brian. Sorry for the late notice, but I've had a really bad afternoon, and I can't meet you for dinner." Yet I couldn't convince myself to place the call. It wasn't just a normal first date; it was a first date on his birthday. Who cancels a date on someone's birthday?

I looked in the mirror. Sobbing had razed all my attempts to look nice. Mascara from one eye was smeared across my cheek; a black swatch of it stuck to the other eyelid. My lips looked like a horizon line, thin and colourless. The ends of my damp hair stuck out. The car, though, was quiet. If I sat in the stillness too long, my thoughts might turn desperate. Images of Holden peeing on the floor and pouring out the polish might swirl around those of my handprint on his butt. That feeling of intense emptiness might return, and I would have another storm to confront.

So I turned the car on and rolled down the window, imagining the breeze blowing away my stress. *Be open to a nice time,* I thought, as I wiped the makeup off with my fingertips. I inhaled, and I exhaled. I put the car in gear and accelerated.

* * *

When I look back on the decision to meet Brian for dinner, I understand its significance. Nothing made sense, and everything felt wrong. I believed my failures. The dissolution of The Plan meant I couldn't know—or trust—the ways I'd survived, and thrived, for so long. I was so close, perhaps closer than I'd ever been before, to letting myself disappear so someone else could trace over the remains of my life.

Brian's correspondence offered a reminder—not of love or desire or escape—but a reminder that possibilities for feeling existed outside of my numb desperation. Even though I reasoned that I couldn't cancel on someone's birthday, I went because Brian reminded me that an evening of conversation, and perhaps a few laughs, could inch me away from the abyss that seemed both close and everlasting.

The second I walked inside the restaurant, Brian saw me and stood up. He wore sky-blue pants and a button-down shirt so close in colour it looked like a suit. Confident colour choices, I thought, and *not* South Dakotan. I smiled and he smiled back, which transformed his face from serious to warm and slightly mischievous.

"How are you?" He pulled out a chair. He was taller than I'd remembered.

"Okay, I guess. I had a really rough afternoon. I should tell you that now," I replied.

"Do you want a drink?" he asked.

"Please," I replied. He made eye contact with the waiter, who hurried over.

"I'd like another martini, please," he told him. "And what would you like?"

"If that's a Cosmo," I said, noticing pink liquid in the bottom of his glass, "I'll have one too." The waiter nodded. Brian turned back to me.

"I like pink cocktails," he said. My giggle mixed with his chuckle and followed the waiter as he turned away.

"Do you want to talk about your rough day?" When he sat back a bit, I noticed his bowtie. Such a nerd, I thought. This common condition stirred my affection.

That evening, our conversation ranged, but I did most of the talking.

Over cocktails: Holden's mystery behaviours and meltdowns. Brian responded with empathy. "Children have a life to build," he said. "Sometimes they really build it on our backs, and it hurts." Although I didn't think he grasped the intensity of what it meant to parent Holden, that he sought common ground for understanding struck me as singular.

Over salad: I unfolded a design I'd done for my garden, four pieces of graph paper I'd plotted out and Scotch-taped together. I pointed out the herb-spiral garden in the middle that Holden and I had built with concrete pavers salvaged from my parents' and neighbours' yards. My finger traced the compost bin, the circles representing the three fruit trees I'd planted, and the wire cages along the back fence for varieties of vegetables that liked to curl around things.

Over braised chicken and pork chops with cherry sauce: We talked about poetry. Brian imagined various ways to inscribe my words in land, from the surface of a sheet of paper to my backyard. I'd never imagined anything quite like it, but I admired how it broke convention. "I could write with a lawn mower," he said. "I think I could step off a stanza and wear the words into the grass. Or I can design an instrument that will inscribe the words." He engaged my work with his own artistic understanding. His architectural thinking impressed me, and I gleaned a sense of the world through his eyes.

Over dessert: We exchanged travel stories. I shared anecdotes about Japan, India, and Italy; Brian described living briefly in Berlin and Dublin. I learned about how many places he'd lived growing up—Ohio, Texas, Canada—and for school—New York and Canada. Each place sparked creative endeavours for both of us.

The date ended rather abruptly. I realized it was almost 7:00, and that I would need to meet Holden soon. Abel was moving into his rental house that weekend, so this would be the last three-hour visit before he'd start spending longer periods of time with him.

"I had a great time tonight," I said as I stood up to go. "Thank you so much for your patience with my wandering conversation." I noticed Brian slip his credit card into the bill pocket for the waiter, and I felt a twinge of guilt about the expensive dinner. I hadn't dated since I was a struggling graduate student. Should I offer to pay? I took out my wallet, but Brian just looked at me with a smile and shook his head no. "I've got this one," he said.

Brian walked me outside to my car, and we shared an awkward goodbye. I wanted to stay and talk, even if it was outside the restaurant, but I didn't want to keep Holden waiting. I waved to Brian and jumped in my car.

I arrived home feeling like myself, stimulated by ideas and stories. Two minutes later, Abel walked Holden to the door and told me that he'd talked to him about his earlier behaviour. When Abel left, Holden's eyes filled with tears. I sat on the couch hugging him.

"You'll see Daddy in two days, Holden. Don't worry," I said. He nodded. After he calmed down, I helped him get ready for bed, read him some books, and tucked him in.

Holden's sadness only dampened my spirits a little. Exhausted but excited, I replayed moments of the date as I drifted off to sleep, wondering what—if anything—would be waiting for me in my inbox the next morning.

* * *

According to Tschumi, if an architect uses the palimpsest as a design strategy, they can add layers from other sources—other cities, other parks, other buildings—to create something new. I imagine a model or a drawing where I can see the layers of the past: a thin outline of a wall, a tangle of pipes just under the ground. Perhaps an altered landscape—a gouge or groove—needs to be engaged by the new design. Perhaps trees or shadows of nearby structures can be used. These are material considerations—the thinking through of elements.

That summer, our courtship unfolded on the ruins of our past marriages. Brian and I exchanged letters, photographs, poem drafts, and architecture sketches punctuated by lunches and occasional dinners when Holden was with his dad. I caught a sense of Brian's romantic side when he brought me a bouquet of sunflowers. I hugged him, pressing my face into his button-down shirt, and inhaled the scents of sweat and patchouli. And I took Brian's traces—his gestures, his words—with me throughout the day and built with them. Sometimes, after dropping Holden off at summer daycare, I took my laptop to Cottonwood, settled into my favourite booth with a mug of chai or a cup of dark roast, and fell into writing.

Our new relationship inspired new work.[4] Sipping my drink, I reread our emails, pondering a photograph, painting, or song that Brian referenced. One image was of the Toledo Museum of Art, whose 360 glass panels mesmerized me. I researched glassmaking and layered that language with a description of the glass pavilion: *Glass begins as flint, sand, or spar—a siliceous substance fused with a flux*.... My own concerns emerged through the lenses of art and artmaking, ending with insight into relationships, *how perfect fusions become puddles of sand* over time. Often, my poems distilled results of our wide-ranging conversations via voice and email. "Didactic" began over a discussion Brian and I had about our approaches to teaching; Brian described learning through haptic inquiry, so I applied this concept to various contexts. A love poem resulted. I sent Brian the opening line, "Throw open the library of your body," and he replied with an image of Titian's *Venus of Urbino*. "The artist finished these paintings with his fingers to give them the texture of the glow of light," Brian wrote.

My final draft of that poem uses images of fingers exploring books and maps as if a lover's body. Our first kiss happened next to a world atlas—the boldly coloured, classroom kind. It hung in Brian's apartment on the wall above his kitchen table. "Russia's still the Soviet Union on this map," he said. I studied the dissolved national boundaries, marvelling at how much can change in such a short time. A few minutes later, I was sorting items from a grocery sack next to the sink when I felt his hand on my shoulder. I turned to meet his lips. That first kiss, short and passionate, swept away any doubts about what kind of relationship we were building.

Brian related to me as an artist, a scholar, and a maker of things. We spoke different dialects of the same language. It didn't surprise me that the intensity of our intellectual exchanges mirrored our physical intimacy as that unfolded. Falling in love with Brian meant falling into love with all of his dimensions.

That summer, still vibrant in my imagination due to its intensity of emotions—the sugar-flinging, nail-polish-pouring, abyss-peering, sunflower-staring—I began to use the palimpsest strategy to move forward with my life without even knowing it. I'd already been using it in writing. Turning words and forms of poetry over in my mind, I knew their meanings and how they held their own traces of history, and yet I appreciated the prisms of colour they cast and how they illuminated insights, sparked connections, and revealed paradoxes. With them, I created new work. The flow of research and writing, which had long sustained me, continued to do so. My creative practice stripped me to my intellectual core—curious, thoughtful, calm; writing demanded only that I pay attention, however fragmented that attention was.

With Brian, I felt the tumble of new love. Sometimes I questioned myself for allowing new love in so quickly after the divorce; sometimes

I marvelled at the feeling of new love and wondered if I was allowed to feel happy at all. I had a changing, challenging child to raise; I had a household to run and a job to hold on to. None of this was part of The Plan, the illusion of which still held power. So I worked on not trying to map out the what-happens-next before it happened. I tried to take it day by day.

My time with Brian centred me and grounded me, much like writing did. He was busy designing an undergraduate curriculum and envisioning a graduate complement; he spent time building materials for studio culture, such as desks and pin-up boards; he supervised his summer student workers; and he invested time in advocating for the new department. Since we didn't have a lot of time together, we made sure most of it could be quality time—lingering over dinner or driving to Sioux Falls for an evening out. Brian didn't compete for my time, attention, or affection; he folded himself into margins.

* * *

In just a few months, I would finally know what caused Holden's meltdowns and tantrums; I'd have a name for what erased his ability to understand what I said to him and use language as he once had. That summer, though, I watched the *process* of the palimpsest at work in him. Something was erasing Holden's skills. Sometimes I thought I could see it happening. In August, we took that trip to western South Dakota—the Badlands, Mount Rushmore, and Rapid City—with my friend from high school and his family. Holden wet his pants twice. He obsessed over controlling a game of putt-putt golf. He ignored the other boys his age. In these moments, I could see traces of what he had once been able to do. The changes rewriting him seemed both dramatic and subtle. I struggled to understand what design the seizures had for Holden—what they were building on the form of my altered boy.

I integrated Brian slowly into Holden's life. Brian met Holden as a dull-eyed child obsessed with *Angry Birds* and *Plants vs. Zombies*. On occasion, Brian could cajole him out of the fog to trace shapes on paper with a Sharpie or watch (and sometimes dance) to Daft Punk's "Around the World." A few times, the three of us met at the playground near Brian's apartment. Holden loved it when Brian pushed him high on the swing. A few times Brian joined us for dinner at our house. When I ask Brian now, years later, what memory of Holden stands out from that summer, he says: "The night I found him with a razor."

My memory of that night is faulty. Perhaps we'd been eating dinner or cleaning up from it. Perhaps Brian had been checking his email on his laptop while I reorganized Holden's busy boxes. Either way, neither of us thought much of it when Holden left the living room and headed toward the bathroom. The toilet flushed. I expected him to walk back out, but after a few minutes when he still hadn't returned, I asked Brian to check on him.

"Christine, you'd better come here," I heard seconds later. I met them both in the bathroom, Holden with a disposable razor in his hand. "He was standing on the toilet trying to see the mirror. It was on his cheek," Brian said. Holden's expression was confused, distant.

"This is dangerous, Holden. What were you doing?" I tried to take the razor from his hand, but he held on to it, his face clouding with anger. Seconds later, though, he let go of the pink handle and walked out of the bathroom in tears.

"What was he thinking? Doesn't he know that's dangerous?" Brian talked through scenarios of what could've happened if we'd waited another minute. "He could've cut himself." The sight of blood nauseated Brian, but Holden's disregard for something dangerous unnerved him profoundly. Brian seemed to understand the need for my vigilance and comprehend Holden's disconnect with logic.

Part of me worried that it would all be too much for Brian, but if Holden's needs ever gave Brian pause early in our courtship, he never told me. That summer, I think he felt sorry for us. He understood how epilepsy shaped our lives, and he felt sad that it took more than it gave, so he respected the space I needed to parent Holden and supported me by listening, troubleshooting, and distracting me when necessary. Today, when I ask Brian why he, someone who hadn't planned to parent any other children besides his daughter, chose to date a woman with a child who needed intense parenting, he doesn't have much of an answer.

With Abel living close by, Brian said that he didn't imagine himself in a parenting role, but more as a bonus adult in Holden's life.

Another part of me wondered if Brian would ever be able to read the palimpsestic conditions through the screens of insomnia and seizures. I wondered if he would even see how Holden moved through the world before the seizures: curious and gregarious and charming. Would he treat him differently if he couldn't? Feel a different set of emotions in regard to him? I didn't know exactly. Maybe not knowing Holden before the seizures started freed him from expectations. Maybe it enabled him to accept Holden as he was not in relationship to plans or dreams. In any case, Brian's understanding of Holden was composed on open ground. What he built with Holden would be new and would be his own.

Chapter Nine

INTERLOCUTION: to speak between

THE HIGHLY ANTICIPATED SECOND-OPINION APPOINTMENT at the University of Minnesota happened at the end of August. After an afternoon of engaging Holden with games, puzzles, and attempts at conversation—all to assess his learning—a neuropsychologist pronounced, "I'm certain I know what this is, and I know a specialist who can help."[1]

"What do you mean, 'this'?" I asked.

"It's a medical issue, so I can't be the one to diagnose him." Even these professionals need other professionals, I thought, stunned yet again. Then his voice became serious. "It's very important we get you in right away. I'll write the referral letter myself." His urgency implied danger, and what he obscured—a name, a treatment plan, a prognosis—sent me reeling. I rubbed my sweaty hands on my skirt when he extended his hand. I shook it but didn't know what more to say beyond thank you. What I felt prickled my skin and was familiar: my body suspended over an abyss, my voice sucked away by fear.

Three weeks later, we were back in the Twin Cities, this time at Children's and General Hospitals in St. Paul. The morning's sequence of checking in, obtaining a badge, learning visitor rules, navigating labyrinthine hallways, and answering questions by both a regular nurse and her assistant confused and exhilarated me. I felt so close to knowing what to name this mystery. Yet at each stage, I had to coax Holden. He was done with doctors, and he wanted to go home. I didn't blame him.

We were watching television in the middle of the children's epilepsy unit when Dr. Jones walked over and introduced himself.

"Holden's room will be ready soon, and then we'll get the EEG leads on. In the meantime, I have some questions." He sat down nearby, and I joined him so we didn't interrupt Holden, who was pleased by the cartoons. Dr. Jones had to ask only one or two questions before I launched into a summary of the past two years. He listened, facing me but observing Holden, too. Finally, I paused. He took a deep breath.

"Have you come across Landau-Kleffner syndrome?" Dr. Jones weighed his words, enunciating each one to give it its full weight of sound and meaning.

"Um, yes, I think so. I mean, I recall that name, but I don't remember much about it," I said. "It was one of the scary ones." A flush of shame rose in my cheeks. The twin toddlers playing cars on the floor sent one careening past our table. I looked up. Another car crashed into the high countertop across the room, behind which three EEG technicians watched monitors. The children squealed with delight.

I turned back to Dr. Jones, trying to find words to respond. I was ashamed because I wasn't telling the whole truth: I knew LKS involved language loss. I was ashamed because I hadn't read enough: there must've been more about LKS that would've made me connect Holden to it. I was ashamed because I hadn't recognized Holden—or refused to—in the symptom list.

"Well, the EEG will tell us for sure." He paused and looked at Holden, still immersed in cartoons.

"I limit his screen time at home," I said, embarrassed by how long he had been watching.

"Most kids with LKS fall into screens," he said. A teenager shuffled out of her room to a desk with a computer, coloured cords trailing past her shoulders and gathering into a black backpack. Other children watched television in their rooms along the periphery of the unit, doors ajar.

"I'll try not to let that happen." I felt defensive even though Dr. Jones hadn't said anything accusatory. I equated screen time with lazy parenting. The shame and guilt manifested in resolution: I promised myself that I would keep Holden engaged with the world—travel, field trips, art, music—in any way possible.

Dr. Jones nodded with an expression that contradicted his affirmation. I suspected that I didn't quite know what I was facing.

"I'll be back tomorrow," he said. Then he turned to Holden to say goodbye to him.

* * *

Dr. Jones confirmed the diagnosis of LKS the next morning. He explained that the disorder looked different in every child, and that other neurologists made distinctions among variants of LKS and a nearly identical syndrome, CSWS, because symptoms overlapped. He preferred to call it all LKS. "I treat each child as an individual based on the EEG and the presenting symptoms—language fluency and academic skills," he said. Although there wasn't a consensus on what caused LKS, specialists believed it was an autoimmune response resulting in pervasive seizure activity that could be seen only on an EEG. This seizure activity was different from the kind that caused convulsions.[2]

Dr. Jones outlined his treatment plan. He ordered an MRI to rule out a lesion or structural problem in the brain itself, and he changed the medication regimen completely. He removed the Valium straight away. (Later I learned that Dr. Porter had started Holden on the right protocol with Valium, but she'd failed to follow up with an EEG three months into the treatment to reassess as the course designed. This error seemed significant because the earlier the treatment, the more time a doctor had to try different methods to arrest the pervasive seizure activity that caused regression and brain damage.) He also prescribed a new anti-epilepsy drug as well as prednisone, a steroid. Prednisone countered the autoimmune-related inflammation in Holden's brain.

"We don't understand how or why it works, just that it does for some children," Dr. Jones said. Due to the side effects of excessive weight gain, mood swings, and bone loss, some neurologists prescribed steroids in large doses for a six-week period and then tapered them, but Dr. Jones preferred smaller doses over longer periods of time.

All this new information affected me. I knew it would take some time before I could take it in—read about it, talk about it. So when Dr. Jones asked me if I had questions, I only managed to squeak one out: "What's Holden's prognosis?"

Dr. Jones sat back. A few seconds slipped by before he spoke.

"I don't have a crystal ball," he said. If the MRI revealed something structurally wrong with Holden's brain, it would mean something different than if seizure activity had a non-structural cause. And sometimes it took experimenting with different medicines to find an effective one. For some children, medication worked, and language returned quite quickly. For others, doctors tried intravenous immunoglobulin therapy—sometimes together with surgery, sometimes not. IVIG therapy used human plasma to treat a wide variety of autoimmune diseases, but it didn't always work with LKS. Neither did multiple subpial transection, a procedure performed by only a select few brain surgeons.[3] These treatments seemed scary, especially since not all of them worked to stop the seizure activity—and no epilepsy specialist seemed to know why some treatments worked for some kids but not for others. For the group of children who didn't respond to medication or weren't candidates for brain surgery, LKS tended to resolve at puberty. Later I would learn what he left out: waiting for this biological shift meant the seizures would have seven or so years to alter Holden's cognitive abilities.

After Dr. Jones left, I sat in Holden's room, my head spinning with half-formed questions. "No crystal ball" wasn't complete, wasn't firm, wasn't satisfactory. I wanted to know Holden's future as sure as I could know my own breath, as I could be certain of my heart thumping in my chest.

Yet a thin sense of relief surfaced too. I knew more. I had the right words.

I began to use them right away. I called Brian first. Hearing his voice calmed me a bit, and I wasn't embarrassed to sputter *Landau-Kleffner syndrome*—the phrase had yet to take root in my mouth. Brian asked a lot of questions. I couldn't answer them, but they informed my inquiry, which unfolded over the next few weeks.

Then I called Abel, summarized the visit, and said I'd follow up when I knew more. I hoped my voice sounded more confident, less vulnerable. When we'd discussed who would attend this appointment, I'd suggested that we could take turns; if there was a follow-up, Abel could take Holden. That was naïve of me; this appointment had been intense. Now I planned to be present at all of them. I wished Abel had been there to learn alongside me, but I also knew that his presence wouldn't have meant we would've approached it as a team.

* * *

In many memoirs written by parents raising children with disabilities, grief follows diagnosis. Sometimes it's brief and fleeting, sometimes it's long and dramatic. Parents grieve their dreams for their children, and they grieve their own imagined lives. In Eva Feder Kittay's *Learning from My Daughter: The Value and Care of Disabled Minds*, she notes this motif as well. When she became a parent of a daughter with significant cognitive disabilities, she also experienced an intense "desire for normalcy" and the grief that accompanies the realization that normalcy is no longer possible. After discussing a few examples, Kittay asks, "The shock, the unravelling of all that you had based your expectations on, the 'terrible news' of abnormality, is immediately comprehensible to most. But why, when the source of the anguish is not death, but abnormality?"[4]

When I landed on this question a decade after Holden's diagnosis, I held it close. It challenged the seemingly ubiquitous association of grief with a change in expectations. Grief wasn't what Holden's diagnosis felt like for me, and it wasn't the emotion it produced. Grief was death's purview. Grief ripped. Grief seared. Grief gripped strong enough to leave one numb and stumbling for days, weeks, years. I'd felt that when Theresa died; I'd watched that happen to my parents. Kittay compelled me to give my emotional state a different name and a different description. Like my understanding of LKS, my words would take time to reveal themselves.

But maybe understanding took more time because no one had yet mentioned disability. Dr. Jones framed it medically: medication, treatment. There was no typical, no usual, no normal for this abnormal. Dr. Jones never used the word *disability*. Perhaps his choice of phrase was euphemistic ("the impact of LKS on 'academic skills'") but that didn't conjure disability either. It's impossible to know for certain how the framework of disability might have changed my experience of this part of Holden's diagnostic journey, but I do know that the concept of disability carried weight. I understood it as a state of being that needed serious time and attention. *Disability* would have meant grappling outright with a significant and difficult alteration of The Plan as opposed to the slow and progressive way I experienced change. Perhaps because my current knowledge of disability gives me so many more tools to support and advocate for Holden, I imagine I could've benefited from a more comprehensive understanding earlier. I might've understood that we would be on this path for a long time, and with that understanding, I could've prepared for a different life.

Instead, Dr. Jones gave me a snapshot of the night sky with the stars as symptoms of LKS. His explanation left me with a vague understanding of how this disorder could affect Holden and with the responsibility of connecting the stars to make sense of it all. I knew Holden's constellation would be unique.

* * *

I began to research LKS before Holden left the hospital, but in 2012 sections about LKS on epilepsy websites were few and far between. I learned that LKS occurs most frequently in children between three and seven years old. Drs. Landau and Kleffner, the first to write about the phenomenon in 1957, noted that the six children under their care began having trouble understanding words for no apparent reason.[5] As I read, I spoke words and phrases from the websites aloud—*auditory agnosia, pure word deafness, aphasia*—as if they were words in a poem, as if hearing them would reveal their meaning. What was a *pure* word? How could one qualify *deafness*?

As Holden lost language, I gained a new one. With definitions, glimmers of understanding grew. *Pure word deafness* meant hearing parts of a word, like the middle or end, but not the whole word. *Aphasia* meant the loss of the ability to express speech. *Auditory agnosia* meant the inability to interpret sounds. They illuminated a few typical conversations I'd had recently with Holden:

"Mom?" Holden asked.

"Right here. Yes?"

"Nothing." He glanced up at me and then back down at his iPad.

"Okay," I said.

"Sorry!" he replied.

"No worries," I said.

"You're welcome."

He knew I was speaking, but he hadn't understood what I'd said. Even though I understood that the interpretation of sound happens in the brain, I pictured swabs of cotton in Holden's ears—some sounds making it through or around the cotton, others muffled. He filled in gaps with answers based on his prior experience. What was lost wasn't the entirety of language—sounds just no longer made sense in the ways they once had.

I also learned that language loss may occur slowly or very quickly and may eventually progress to mutism.[6] Children may also appear to be autistic or developmentally delayed, although intelligence usually appears to be unaffected. Communication problems may lead to behavioural or psychological disorders such as hyperactivity, aggressiveness, and depression. These facts explained why I had trouble seeing Holden's odd communication as language loss and why his fluctuating abilities were difficult to plot; they were part of the disorder. In this context, behavioural problems connected seizure activity to episodes of pouring nail polish onto the floor and trying to eat shards of glass.

Once home, I pored over research that I found in medical databases using my university credentials. I never fully comprehended the medical jargon, but I learned explanations for why Holden's language was affected:

"persistent convulsive discharges in brain tissue largely concerned with language communication result in the functional ablation of these areas."[7] I looked up the definitions of words: *ablation*—a reduction in volume; *functional ablation* meant seizures left the areas used to process language unworkable. And the reason the seizure activity caused interference in Holden's ability to process language and speak (even when he wasn't actively seizing) was that disturbances caused a loss of the ability to process complex auditory signals.

I'd witnessed evidence, but now I had names for the happenings. Now I could circle the brightest stars on the snapshot—Holden's night sky.

Echolalia, "sounds imitated without expressive awareness,"[8] explained the *Mini Ninjas* episode. One evening as we were finishing dinner, Holden got up to use the bathroom. Two minutes later, I heard, "Mom! I want to play *Mini Ninjas*!" I put down my fork and rounded the corner as the toilet flushed. Holden walked out of the bathroom with his jeans around his ankles. "I want to play *Mini Ninjas*! I want to play *Mini Ninjas. Mini Ninjas*!"

"Okay. Pull up—"

"I want to play *Mini Ninjas.*" Holden had a blank look on his face, eyes and cheeks relaxed. He pulled up his pants, and I followed him down the hall. "I want to play *Mini Ninjas.*" He looked around the living room, as if searching for actual ninjas, and plopped down on the couch. "I want to play *Mini Ninjas.*"

"We don't have that—"

"Mom! I want to play *Mini Ninjas*!" He looked at me, brows furrowed.

"I'm not sure what you mean, Holden," I said. He seemed to be talking in code. I inventoried my associations: *Mini Ninjas* was a video game we didn't own. Did he want to play it? Or another video game? Did he want to play *Banzai Blade* on the iPad? Or did he want to play with a ninja-like toy—a sword, perhaps? Or perhaps dress up in a ninja costume? Maybe he wanted to read *Yoshi's Feast* because a character resembled a ninja. He had the actual *Mini Ninja* game at Abel's house; perhaps he wanted to go there? Each time I suggested one of these possibilities, Holden repeated the declaration as if he were a student studying for an exam or an actor rehearsing nuances of a memorized line.

Then he spied *Green Eggs and Ham* on the floor and opened the book. "I want to play *Mini Ninjas*. I want to play *Mini Ninjas*. Oh. *Sam I am, that Sam I am, I do not like green eggs and ham ...*" Holden flipped through a few pages. No more ninjas.

Despite the definition of echolalia, I reasoned *mini ninja* could hold meaning; it seemed Holden couldn't find the right words to communicate his intent. Later, Holden's neuropsychologist would address communication in her report: "Holden's tendency to repeat the last word or phrase as he has heard it is likely, at least in part, representative of his attempt to comprehend and engage in a conversation, and should be treated as such. However, it should not be assumed that Holden has understood what was said if he is able to repeat the last word."[9] *Another reason I shouldn't assume his speech was devoid of meaning just because I couldn't decipher it*, I thought.

Creating new words—*neologisms*—was another bright-star symptom. As someone intimate with figurative language, I noticed Holden's new words as well as how he made metaphoric associations similar to neologisms. At SDSU's homecoming, Holden and I donned our blue and yellow Jackrabbit sweatshirts and found a spot in front of Cottonwood Café to watch the parade. We sipped hot cocoa between our cheers for the marching bands, the swirl of music surrounding us. Holden collected a bag of Tootsie Rolls, lollipops, Pixy Stix, and bubble gum thrown to him from the students on the floats. Afterward, as we walked down the sidewalk, Holden held up his bag and exclaimed a synecdoche: "That was a great candy store!"

Other neologisms began to pop up, too. After I showed Holden a prairie landscape video, wind howling, he'd replied, "I hear the dust." At the store, he'd paused before baskets of peppers in the produce aisle: "Look! Hotchiladas!" How Holden put those words together to convey his pleasure and observations amused me. In my writerly world, coining new words, creating metaphors, and mixing senses to make fresh imagery were achievements. For Holden, they signalled a breakdown in language use. One evening he saw our dinner of rice and stir-fried shrimp, then pointed to the Sriracha—rooster emblazoned on the bottle—and exclaimed, "Cockadoodle spicy!" Delight swept over me even as I knew the next moment he could be grasping for words.

* * *

Kittay writes that disability is a relational trait: "a misfit between one's body (or mind) and the physical and social environment."[10] Simple, yet capacious. Had I known this earlier, I would have seen all the symptoms as manifestations of misfit along a continuum that ranged from a slim gap to a chasm, from easy to impossible to adapt to. Her words would have given me a host of ways to think about how my life as Holden's mom had changed, was changing, would change. Had I known about her research and experience—her assertion that "disability can involve a reorientation toward life that can be neutral or positive"[11]—I would have had a clear, solid framework with which to work.

Although I didn't yet have the word, I sensed it. I knew that I was moving in a new direction, that my perspective was profoundly shifting. It felt like the first week I lived in Türkiye, apprehending the depth of learning I would acquire as a result of living there for two years. It felt like revision in writing, insight unfurling as I understood the fresh direction for a poem, essay, or project. This sense blended excitement, as I was enticed by the new, and resistance, as I knew the time and intense focus I would need to accomplish the work.

Without having the word for it, I was reorienting my life, and I would need to reorientate it more. Not grieving and no longer desperate, I felt the pull of the abyss vanish for me—but I think it opened for Holden.

Although not mentioned in many of the websites or journal articles as a symptom, Holden appeared depressed. Where once I wondered how I could see depression in a child, I now knew. At least once every other day, Holden wept. He'd sit at the kitchen counter, feet dangling from the stool, his eyes glazing over. Then his lids relaxed, bottom lip pushed out. His fist rubbed out tears. I imagined these episodes stemmed from sheer exhaustion, exhaustion from the work of understanding, the work of finding words, or the work of reacting to the medications he popped into his mouth twice a day. I wondered if he missed his dad, but he saw him often; I felt this reason was only part of the picture. Holden hurt in a way he couldn't explain, but I explained it as depression.

When he wept, he cried in silence until his tears dried up.

Sometimes he cried the length of a shower, as showers had started to scare him. Perhaps once he had turned the knob (or I had, by accident), forgetting what would happen—and the water got too hot or too cold. He never got burned, but maybe the temperature shift was enough. Perhaps he hated the sensation of the water on his skin. Perhaps a shower took him away from his favourite thing, his iPad. He had to bathe, though. During tearful showers, his muscles relaxed. Yet he still cried. I shampooed his hair gently, remembering how much I loved it when my grandmother washed my hair when I was his age. I wondered if it gave him comfort.

Sometimes the episode lasted the length of a meal of quesadillas and applesauce. He nibbled a triangle of quesadilla; he spooned applesauce into his mouth. The tears still fell.

Sometimes he cried the length of a shopping trip. His snow pants and winter coat filled the cart. Knees to chest, he took off his knit cap, tears streaming down his cheeks. "What's wrong, Holden?" I'd ask. "Do you want Goldfish? Froot Loops?" No response. "Let's go look at the lobsters!" Distraction didn't work, and he rarely answered during meltdowns anyway. Without a solution, I offered comfort by rubbing his back or hugging him. Even though I could see depression and name it as a star in Holden's LKS constellation, I didn't know what I could do about it beyond my attempts to show him I cared.

* * *

The autumn of 2012, while I waited to see whether Dr. Jones's new treatment would work, I adjusted my routines to better support Holden. He needed constant supervision, day and night. By mid-autumn—whether due to increased seizure activity, the side effects of steroids, or the absence of Valium—insomnia increased. Once or twice per night, Holden got up ready to start the day. I curled up alongside him in bed, hoping he'd relax and drift off to sleep. I always did, but then I'd startle awake to find him playing with toys. Sometimes he wanted to watch a video or play with his iPad or dump out toy bins. After a couple of hours, he'd fall back to sleep. This happened several nights each week, yet he didn't sleep in or nap during the day.

Caffeine helped me counter my sleep deprivation, and when Holden was at his dad's, I slept longer and deeper. But that changed when I told Dr. Jones's nurse about Holden's trouble sleeping. They suggested that he sleep at home every night during the school week instead of at his dad's, so instead of keeping him there half the week, Abel brought him home before bedtime during the week. That meant he stayed only one weekend night at his dad's.

To be in closer proximity to Holden at all times, I moved my toiletries from the downstairs bathroom where I usually showered to the bathroom upstairs, so I'd be more likely to hear him wake up and start moving about the house. I showered as soon as I woke up so I could do so while he still slept—at least, in theory. Worried that he'd get up in the middle of the night and not make enough noise to rouse me, I added locks to the front door and the sliding door to the basement so he couldn't easily get downstairs, into the garage, or onto the porch. When Holden was with his dad, I worked more intensely to make up for time lost. My productivity habit—following a daily schedule—no longer worked. I had little control over my day when Holden was in my care; routine could be upended by a meltdown or tantrum or aimless wandering around the house.

Every day, I tried to get Holden to laugh at least once. Sometimes I tickled him a bit to accomplish that. I tried to provide him with activities he had liked in the past, even if they failed to engage him or a meltdown prevented us from finishing them. One morning that autumn when my mom visited, he made a recycled robot out of household materials with her. She did most of the work, but he helped glue the materials together and seemed to enjoy the activity. One Sunday, Brian and I took him to the Great Plains Zoo in Sioux Falls, and although he spent most of the time running from exhibit to exhibit with nary a glance at the animals, the red panda intrigued him for a good fifteen minutes.

And I still tried to communicate with Holden even though he had stopped using language in any way besides echolalic speech. I still asked him questions. I still gave him directions. I still cracked jokes and acted silly. And because sometimes words did make it through the fog in his brain, I developed a check to see whether he understood me.

"Do you want a kitten?" I'd ask.

"No," he'd respond.

"Chocolate candy bar?"

"No."

"Trip to Disneyland?"

"No."

"What do you want?"

"I don't want to talk about it."

If he responded "yes," something was getting through. "No" was his safe answer; it often maintained the status quo.

When words failed, I used touch to communicate my love. Often I sat next to Holden on the couch and hugged him, wrapping my arms around him fully. Or, if he was playing a video game or watching television, I cuddled with him and ran my hand through his hair. Sometimes I just sat next to him as I worked. I wanted my presence to communicate how much I cherished him as my child, but there was more than that. Our proximity also helped me anticipate his wants and needs. Kittay describes this aspect of caregiving as an ethic component of care, which she defines as tripartite: as labour, as an attitude (or disposition), and as a virtue. She writes: "The attentive responsiveness critical to successful caring is made possible—often, at least—by an empathetic connection to and understanding of the other. These enable us to 'read' the mind of another, especially in cases where the other is either temporarily or permanently incapable of communicating through speech."[12] I'd begun to develop this attentive responsiveness, although I didn't have Kittay's framework yet.

One evening, I turned to study Holden's face as he watched cartoons. He was such a beautiful boy, getting the best features from both the Stewart and the Nuñez families. Slightly cleft chin. Deep eyes. Sometimes his eyes flicked with expectation or his lips twitched with amusement. He seemed sleep-deprived, which made me wonder why he didn't just sleep. He seemed detached from the world and nearly all desire. I breathed in the intensity of his silence, ghosts of words he once could say dissolving into the air.

I recalled the day after his birth—a thirty-hour labour that ended with a C-section—when the wind had whistled across the hospital parking lot and slammed into windows. I was adrift in the fuzz of sleep deprivation and the blur of hormone overload when he cried his alarm-clock cry. My milk let down and began to stream from my tingling nipples. My heart quickened, not because my body was working in new ways or because my soaked gown embarrassed me or because Holden's need shocked me, but because my post-surgery state kept me from reaching him in his bassinet. It took three minutes for the nurse to arrive, loosen his swaddling, and hand him to me. He latched. As milk passed from my body to his, the room's walls, cabinets, and bed blurred. In that space just beyond my skin, Holden and I were anchored. His belly filled and the wind slowed. Then we slept.[13]

Just as we were that day, the two of us were anchored with the world spinning around us. But this world felt different—not just new but unknowable and in constant flux. The understanding that would propel me from day to day wasn't that of implicit trust in The Plan. It meant recognizing that I needed tools to adjust to transitions just as Holden did. He needed me to be flexible and fluid far more than any other person or situation had demanded of me before.

I reached out my hand and brushed Holden's hair to the side. Then I held him, wanting the language of closeness to speak. I wanted him to understand how much I was trying to revise my life—my very way of being in the world—so I could be a better mom for him. I wanted him to know he could count on me—even when I slipped a bit and yelled during one of his tantrums. I wanted him to feel unconditionally loved.

I wish I could write that, as I reoriented, I challenged the "nomenclature of disability" that Kittay argues is built into our vocabulary. I wish I could say I was adapting to new possibilities instead of coping, but at this point I couldn't see them. I wish I could report that I was consciously recalibrating and deliberately learning new skills to challenge cultural narratives about disability. These shifts were underway even though I didn't have those words. I began to draw and redraw lines between the stars in Holden's LKS constellation. I wondered whether they'd shimmer into some kind of sense, perhaps direct me somehow. I felt at the mercy of Holden's brain and how it constantly changed the patterns of our lives and upended basic routines. I had no way to anticipate the fluctuations.

There was no narrative, no what-happens-next. I had to manage complex weather—a new front moving in multiple times per day—and be ready to react. Most days ended in sublime exhaustion—the mental, emotional, physical, spiritual consequence of constantly adapting.

Chapter Ten

INTERICTAL: occurring between seizures

TWO WEEKS BEFORE CHRISTMAS AND ONE MONTH BEFORE Holden's seventh birthday, I was gathering his school items when, out of the corner of my eye, I saw him stop moving.

"Get back, fuzzy mirror," he said. I thought of the garland we'd pinned around our front door. Turning around, I saw his finger pointing to the blank wall. He stepped backward and his legs crumpled. A clinical seizure.

On the carpet, I rolled him onto his left side. His left hand opened and closed as if he were squeezing a stress ball. "Hap-py. Birth-day," he sang in a breathy voice. Earlier, we'd made a birthday video for my mom, Holden mumbling along and smiling.

When his eyes rolled to the side and locked, I started counting. "One. Two. Three ..." I counted out loud, so that I wouldn't lose track. "Twenty. Twenty-one ..." It had been over a year since he'd had a seizure this big. I rubbed his shoulder through his shirt. No change in his eyes.

"Forty-four. Forty-five." I studied his jaw: clenched or locked? Was his stomach heaving?

"Sixty-seven. Sixty-eight." By 180, I'd have to leave him to get the Diastat. "Seventy-eight. Seventy-nine." The sunlight reflecting off the snow outside illuminated his face. His cheeks hadn't been this full since babyhood. I wondered if it was the prednisone. Around 100, Holden's hand stopped twitching. At 110, his face relaxed.

"You're going to be fine," I said, exhaling fully. I hugged him. After a few more seconds, Holden began to move his arms and legs. His pants were still dry. He grabbed my arm, steadied himself, and crawled onto his bed. I tucked the covers around him. He hugged his teddy bear, Oval, with one arm and closed his eyes.

I sat next to his bed and initiated the post-seizure report calls to Holden's school, Holden's dad, and Holden's neurologist. No one answered, so I left messages. Adrenaline lingered in my body. I'd responded to a seizure on my own and hadn't panicked. I held this sense of accomplishment alongside the fear it rekindled: even with the new protocols, intense seizures were still possible. I wondered again whether the medicine was working, and I wondered, again, whether medicine would ever work. I felt the familiar waves of worry as I watched Holden's peaceful face. I imagined, naively, that sleep helped his brain recover.

* * *

A week after the seizure, on Holden's second visit to St. Paul Children's Hospital for an overnight EEG, I learned seizures—invisible to me—disturbed his sleep. The EEG revealed how often during the night Holden woke up and stayed awake—for nearly an hour or two each time—and it even recorded two larger seizures that didn't wake him up. Even more disappointing, the EEG showed Dr. Jones that the three-month prednisone trial hadn't changed the subclinical seizure activity. At all. Zip. Zero. But Dr. Jones insisted on an EEG every three months for exactly this reason—to gather data to inform his treatment plan. He increased the prednisone frequency to twice per week and added Topamax, another anti-seizure medication.

It had been months since I'd seen my son consistently happy or content. I longed to see the Holden who loved to play and laugh. Since it was Christmastime, I tried to communicate the magic of the season. I read *The Night Before Christmas* to him almost every night for a week, but on Christmas Eve he didn't seem to remember any details, and even though he sat still for the story, his eyes didn't perk up. Even though we'd eaten Grandma's cinnamon rolls every Christmas morning since he was born, Holden sniffed them with disinterest. And he didn't seem to remember what to do with the wrapped gifts with his name on them. When I tore them open, he smiled but quickly lost interest. When family and friends gathered at my parents' home for celebrations, he ran to his room.

Perhaps the increase in steroids heightened his emotions. Perhaps they lengthened his meltdowns and intensified the tantrums. Or perhaps these were signs of further regression. The behaviour seemed a visible manifestation of the seizure activity.

The day after Christmas, Holden and I met some friends in the food court at an upscale mall. As we caught up, I monitored Holden's eating; I needed to time his last bite with giving him his iPad. When Dr. Jones had told me kids with LKS tend to "fall into screens," I vowed that Holden wouldn't. Now I encouraged it. Holden could no longer entertain himself with his own thoughts or join a conversation. He wouldn't colour or look at books on his own. Without a screen to watch videos or play games, he fidgeted and whined.

As he pushed away the tray, I handed him his iPad. He propped up the new screen, complete with a life-proof cover, and launched one angry bird after another into a pyramid of quirky pigs. I talked to my friends for another twenty minutes. When it was time to say goodbye, however, Holden had other ideas.

"I'm. Not. Going!" He spit his words out one at a time.

"We're going back to Grandma and Grandpa's house," I said.

"NO!" He slumped over in the booth.

"Hey, you guys. It was good to see you," I turned to my friend and her daughter. They hadn't seen this version of Holden, even though I'd tried to explain what might happen. We hugged and waved goodbye.

"Let's put the iPad away so we can go to the car." I planned to touch the iPad, point to my bag, and point to my car keys to illustrate. But as I reached out, Holden yanked the iPad away and kicked me in the knee. A dull throb of pain emanated from the point of contact, yet my mind reacted as if he'd broken my patella. I grabbed the iPad, and because he wasn't expecting that, it slipped right out of his hands.

"NO!" He screamed as if I'd hit him. The thought of doing so flashed through my mind but moved right on through. He lunged for the iPad. I stepped back. His body, expecting contact with mine, stumbled forward. Unhinged, he bolted.

I picked up my purse and followed. "Wait, Holden. Slow down." I grabbed his shoulder, but he broke free and began to run, finally stopping near Auntie Anne's pretzel shop. "Come on, Holden," I said. "Let's go to Grandma and Grandpa's." He turned right, walked a few steps, then crumpled to the floor in tears. When I grasped his hand to help him up, he yanked it away.

"NO!" He scooted back a few feet and covered his mouth with his hands. Tears flowed faster now.

Shoppers stared at us: kid in a striped shirt and blue pants sporting a knitted triceratops hat; woman in jeans and a heavy sweater sitting cross-legged in front of him. I rehearsed the narratives I'd developed to explain Holden's behaviour: "Holden's brain works differently than other kids' brains"; "He's got a communication disorder"; "He has a rare form of epilepsy that affects language, memory, sleep, and behaviour." I had one snappy comeback for folks who glared but hadn't used it yet: "My child has an abnormal brain; what's your excuse for rude behaviour?"

I took out my phone. A recording could help doctors see this new level of behaviour. Or could explain to police how this whole episode started. I feared someone would accuse me of child endangerment, so a screen could help me, too.

"This is his fifth or sixth meltdown of the day, even though we've only been out a few hours," I said on the recording. "He won't let me touch him." Shoulders hunched, Holden's crying turned into a forced cry. He wiped his tears off his face. "Can you talk to me now?" I asked.

"NO!" He reached over his body to punch me with his right fist and kick me with his left boot. Then he shoved me, spitting on me as my body moved away from his.

"Why are you kicking me?" He turned away. "Can you find your words?" I asked him three times. For whom was I repeating it? For him, in case it got through? To an audience, in case there was one behind us?

Kicking. Punching. Pushing. Spitting. None were new but all were more frequent. Two weeks before, he hadn't wanted me to turn down the volume on his iPad, so he'd hurled the charger at me; the impact left a welt on my back. I found it difficult to know exactly what to do when Holden seemed aggressive, and no one I asked did either. Sometimes I yelled and threatened. Sometimes I pinned his arms and legs so he couldn't hit or kick me. Sometimes I moved in to hug him, hoping it would defuse his anger. Sometimes I got punched anyway. Sometimes I ushered him into his room to tantrum. If he didn't calm down right away, he usually threw books, toys, and puzzle boxes. In the privacy of our home, it was easier to maintain reason and patience and composure. I could walk away for a minute. I could hold my head in my hands. I could talk out loud and soothe myself far more openly.

Public tantrums added the terror of humiliation and evaluation—someone judging my child and judging me for the way I handled the situation. But it was worse with the physical elements. In hindsight, I wish I could have shifted my attitude and just thought, "Who gives a shit about what anybody thinks?" That would eventually happen, but this was too new, my emotions too prone to ping from bewilderment to anger to fear. I tried to pretend we were alone in the mall, the hundreds of post-holiday shoppers disappearing into thin air. *Just focus on Holden,* I told myself. *It's just him that matters.*[1]

"Can I give you a piggyback ride to the car?" I asked. Anything to exit peacefully.

He turned around the second time I asked, his eyes still teary and puffy. He chewed on his fingertips. He shook his head no.

"Can I get you a treat? Holden, are you hungry?" He turned his back to me again but gazed in the direction of Auntie Anne's. I assumed he was staring; he'd been spacing out for five to fifteen seconds several times a day. I ended the video there. After a few more minutes, I curled my arms around his shoulders without him screaming and pulled him up by his armpits. Hand in hand, we walked to the car in silence.[2]

* * *

In the memoirs I've read by parents raising children with disabilities, the reorientation of their lives occurs in varying degrees of awareness and action across time.[3] Sometimes profound change renders parents unable to reflect until years later, or time-intensive caregiving equates to months passing by without much thought about what it all might mean. Looking back on the winter following Holden's LKS diagnosis, I'm struck by how radically isolated I felt, despite my new knowledge of LKS, my burgeoning relationship with Brian, and the emotional support of my parents and brother—albeit from afar.

Part of what contributed to my isolation was the non-apparent nature of Holden's disability, a combination of the invisible seizures alongside the visible (clinical) ones. Invisibility as a concept can frame several aspects of how people experience disability. Susannah Mintz uses the term to describe "diseases, conditions, and sensations that cannot be observed externally,"[4] such as epilepsy. For Holden, the possibility of clinical seizures, like the one I witnessed before Christmas, as well as the ones visible only on the EEG, added to the complexity of his neurological impairment. As Mintz argues, "invisible disabilities present unique challenges in a society already prone to suspicion about the reality status of illness and provoked to anxiety by incapacity and pain."[5] No one observing Holden sipping his Sprite in the mall would think of him as disabled; a stranger would most likely attribute his meltdown to behavioural issues I couldn't manage.

My struggle to address Holden's behaviour, especially in public but certainly at home as well, underscores the invisible sources of stress and strain that characterize this kind of intense parenting. Because the methods and stories about this kind of parenting were not explicitly part of how I learned to be a parent, these challenges felt like mine alone. Perhaps it's typical, even stereotypical, to admit to feeling isolated as a parent of a disabled child, but this feeling can also be explained by ableism.

Mintz argues that the absence of disability "from the conversations and activities that establish the way a society functions, encompassing social relationships, intellectual and artistic work, and politics"[6] is another way society marginalizes disability experiences. Certainly, complex and diverse stories by people living with bodymind differences were invisible to me. I knew disability only as slices of story, fragments of images, and vague impressions. Disability meant names of diseases and conditions, words and phrases that carried stigma and harmful stereotypes. Without the full language for disability, I couldn't find my experience reflected in wider conversations, let alone begin to articulate it in the context of systemic social structures.

In hindsight, I understand my own isolation, but I am equally frustrated by my slowness. Why did it take me so long to put the pieces of evidence together in a way that made Holden's disability legible to me? By that December's seizure, visit to Dr. Jones, and mall meltdown, I'd already accumulated what should have been sufficient evidence. And some of the best data had been given to me by Dr. Jones's associate, Dr. Pratt.

* * *

I met Dr. Pratt, a neuropsychologist, at Holden's first visit to St. Paul Children's Hospital in September 2012. Dr. Jones introduced me to her as the specialist who could test Holden's learning; even after the EEG pointed to LKS, he wanted a baseline from which to measure Holden's regression or progression in terms of his academic skills. Dr. Pratt gave Holden the requisite cognitive tests, but she also conferred with us about LKS more generally. She excelled at answering questions and never appeared rushed. Her analysis of the taco shop video from the grocery store, for example, provided important insight—a clue I could've read as signalling disability.

"I don't understand what was happening here," I said to her as we sat in Holden's hospital room. I held my phone out for the duration of the clip. She watched and listened, then adjusted a bit in her chair before speaking.

"With LKS, some days or moments of the day are better than others," she said. "The video shows a typical sort of behaviour with LKS. Before the meltdown, he probably didn't understand what you were asking him, and he probably couldn't find the words to tell you what he felt."

"Well, then, in the store, why didn't he just go to the bathroom? Why did he just keep saying taco shop?" I'd asked. "He'd used that bathroom before, and I pointed to the door."

"I don't know exactly, but I look at it this way: in that moment, he simply couldn't." She sat back in her chair. That sentence hung in the air.

He couldn't. Not chose to or chose not to. Simply couldn't.

For nearly two years, every professional I'd come into contact with—Helen, Dr. Porter, the district psychologist—insisted that the solution to Holden's behaviour issues was the application of behaviourist methods. All I needed to do was motivate Holden so he would choose better behaviours. But this model doesn't work for someone who isn't able to choose in particular contexts. The hitting and spitting weren't Holden's fault. These outbursts didn't indicate a lack of good choices or proper motivation. They weren't indicative of an inner moral flaw.

In her report from the first visit, Dr. Pratt wrote: "Holden does also have intermittent generalized epileptiform bursts during wakefulness, which will continue to impact his daily functioning.... Holden will not be able to consistently follow directions, and this should be interpreted in the context of impaired comprehension, rather than 'naughty' or defiant behaviour."[7] She was the first and only professional who had explained it this way. Aside from Holden lashing out because he couldn't express himself appropriately, I hadn't been able to explain the link between LKS and these behaviours. Over time, however, I began to understand the causal relationship between seizure activity and the aggressive responses that Dr. Pratt noted in her report. The seizure activity disrupted Holden's ability to think through complex situations. It took him longer to reach reasonable responses, so I often witnessed the knee-jerk, emotional response—the kind I often feel but can work through and tamp down.

Another clue was Dr. Pratt's comment regarding rigidity—Holden's outbursts during moments of transition. Holden usually moved between a foggy detachment from his context and a fixation on screens. Transitions comprised a myriad of at-home and out-and-about activities: moving from couch to car, home to school, Walmart toy aisle to paper supply section; switching from one television show to another, from tennis shoes to snow boots, from beanbag to bed; changing flavour of Gatorade, brand of granola bar, type of bagel. Some transitions ended in meltdowns or tantrums, but since they appeared random to me, I wasn't sure what sparked them. Holden's iPad often ensured smooth transitions, but sometimes it simply didn't.

So why didn't these clues lead me to naming Holden's intellectual disability explicitly? Why didn't I frame Holden's loss of complex thinking skills—the abilities to wonder, strategize, imagine—as cognitive impairment?[8] Perhaps because, just as with the symptoms of language loss before his LKS diagnosis, Holden was presenting me with evidence for which I didn't yet have a full understanding. Perhaps because I wasn't yet comprehending that Holden wasn't going to return to the trajectory of his life as it had been before the seizures began. I believed that intellectual disability was permanent and obvious; I didn't understand it as invisible, fluid, contextual. I embraced rigid thinking that checked mental boxes such as "can do" or "can't do."

My observations regarding Holden's ability to think through information never conclusively checked the "can't do" box. Because the seizure activity generated a fog of silence, it only seemed that my son couldn't speak or couldn't hear *sometimes*. He only seemed lost inside himself *sometimes*; when the fog thinned, Holden's eyes sparkled again and words came back. Examples of "can do" sprinkled themselves over weeks of time. One afternoon, as we walked toward the grocery store, Holden pointed to a dog that looked like my parents' dog: "There's Sady," Holden said. "That dog looks like Sady. Because Sady is a *schnauzer*." I marvelled how he summoned that word: schnauzer. The experience felt surreal, magical. Holden's fluctuating abilities suggested that his cognitive abilities weren't gone, just trapped.

Another example that checked the "can do" box occurred one evening during our bath-time routine. Holden often screamed at the beginning of a shower, relaxing only after the water had been on for a minute or two. I was helping him put on his pajamas after a long crying spell when he sat down on the closed toilet seat and said, "I'm such an idiot. You don't deserve that." I was shocked. Holden rarely—if ever—put sentences together like that. Sometimes he'd say a word like "idiot," but he'd say it with the intonation from the movie or television show he'd heard it in. This was in his own voice. And he washed his hands and brushed his teeth without prompting. Words plus action made me take what he said seriously; he felt remorse. I felt stunned by this window into his mind. It was so rare to see him name his emotions, let alone reflect on them. Certainly this meant the ability was still in there somewhere.

But perhaps another reason I didn't use the word *disability* was because no one else had yet—at least, no one with authority. Sometimes I wonder if Dr. Jones and Dr. Pratt avoided using *intellectual disability* because they didn't want these words to trap me—and, by extension, Holden—with assumptions, with limitations, with society's dominant narratives of disability as defective and permanent. On one hand, I can see why. Recently, I saw a parent on the LKS/CSWS discussion board refer to her ten-year-old son as her "forever baby." With active seizure activity not changed by medication, she assumed he'd always be non-verbal, and she read that as a reason to frame him as a baby. Other families affirmed her perspective. Might her belief that he would always be a baby mean she wouldn't advocate for him in school? Might it mean she would choose to leave any academic pursuits off the table because infants don't need an education?

On more than one occasion, Dr. Jones resisted giving a prognosis and warned against self-fulfilling expectations. When I see parents like this one on the discussion board, I can see Dr. Jones's wisdom. Because this disorder is in flux, locking down a future may limit the child's potential. On the other hand, this line of thinking perpetuates the invisibility of disability.[9]

* * *

If reorienting my life to parenting a child with a disability generated extreme emotional responses in me, reorienting his life to a seizure-shaped consciousness did the same for Holden. By his third visit to see Dr. Jones, Holden's feelings signalled a deepening fear and despair.

We were standing on the sidewalk in St. Paul, Minnesota. Workers had shovelled the six inches of snow into piles—an April snow that had started in Brookings the afternoon before and followed us to St. Paul. The thick, wet snow made for horrible driving conditions. I'd planned to leave Brookings just as the storm started, but I stalled, hoping its trajectory would change. Rescheduling meant waiting another six weeks, and Holden's language and behaviours were worsening. I'd read enough about regressions to know that a more severe language loss could mean mutism. It could mean he would lose his ability to use the toilet, and he could also lose the moments of clarity I saw pass over his face a few times a day. I hoped Dr. Jones had more ideas for ways to tackle LKS beyond the medication changes he'd already made.

Too scared to drive alone but too scared to miss the appointment, I called Brian. He drove us through the night to St. Paul, then turned around and drove back to Brookings so he could teach. My mom said she'd drive up to St. Paul the next day and drive us back to Brookings when the roads cleared.

"Holden, we're going to see Dr. Jones now," I said, pointing at the hospital entrance. Holden's gaze followed my arm.

"No!" He pitched himself into a pile of snow, face down. I squatted and grabbed his snowsuit. Weighed down by our bags, I teetered for a second, then pulled him up and out. His face was reddened from the snow.

Checking in didn't get easier. I wheelchaired Holden to the pediatric epilepsy unit because he refused to walk. Then, after a two-hour check-in, health update, and lunch of cheese quesadilla, the EEG tech walked in with the cart. Holden let out a plaintive "Nooooooo." I scooched onto the bed and held his hand.

"Hey, man. It's okay. It won't hurt," the tech said, adjusting the bed's position. The tech's voice held a trace of an accent—Caribbean, perhaps. Holden looked at him and nodded. Holden watched him organize the marker, washable glue, and sensors. But as the tech moved to a position at the top of the bed, Holden twisted around to watch him. No soothing words, no reminders that Holden had done this before helped. Eventually, the tech left and came back with another tech, two nurses in purple scrubs and colourful Danskos, and a nursing assistant who planted herself in the corner of the room. We tried to distract Holden with his iPad and cartoons and singing and logic; he twisted away from the tech and thrashed in the bed. We surrounded him, holding down his arms and legs, hoping he'd realize that it didn't hurt. He batted us away. The professionals didn't seem angry or surprised, but I was worried *and* surprised. He'd had so many EEGs before. They didn't hurt. What was going on? Why now?

The nursing assistant disappeared and reappeared with a surfboard-shaped object covered in Velcro-laced fabric. It was bright blue.

"We're going to need to secure him. It'll make it go faster," a nurse told me. I nodded yes but looked away. I didn't want her to see my disappointment; nothing I did worked to calm him down.

"We're going to wrap you up in this, like a burrito," she told Holden. It took two seconds. *I wonder if it feels like a straitjacket*, I thought. My disappointment in myself melted into pain. Holden cried the whole time the tech worked—at lightning speed—to get the electrodes on. I cued up "Life's a Happy Song" on my phone because Holden liked it so much, but he kept crying. When all the leads were secured, they removed the restraints.

What was Holden thinking as they did this? He seemed profoundly sad. I recalled being a sick child with a deep cough that kept me up at night. Mom tried to put some Vicks VapoRub on my chest. When I pushed away her hand, she had Theresa hold me down while she applied it. I can still feel the sticky, smelly stuff and the way my shoulders squirmed while Theresa pinned my arms. Afterwards, when the guck stuck to my shirt, I felt an innocent hatred toward my mom and sister. That feeling vanished, but I remember the event viscerally. Would Holden feel harmed by this? His cries told me that his body would remember, even if epilepsy wiped the memory away.

* * *

During that visit, Dr. Pratt dropped by again to test Holden's learning. She wanted to see whether his skills had slipped. On the first visit, she'd completed an initial academic and language assessment to serve as a diagnostic tool for LKS as well as establish a baseline for future progress or regression. This test was nearly identical to the first one.

She sat on the side of Holden's bed and arranged a few sets of spiral-bound images, puzzles, and a notebook. She explained that since LKS caused a child's language ability to fluctuate, she needed to ask questions in a particular order. Then she flipped to the first page in a book, which featured a pig, a horse, and a cow.

"What is the animal that gives milk?" She asked. Holden pointed to the cow. "Good." She flipped to the next page. "What do people use to cut paper?"

"Scissors!" Holden said, pointing to the scissors.

"Good!" A variety of kitchen items decorated the next page. "What do people use to eat food?" Holden blinked. *Point to the fork!* I thought. He held up his hand but hesitated.

"What do you use to eat, Holden?" I asked. He glanced at me, then returned to the picture. When he still didn't point, Dr. Pratt turned to the next page and asked him a similar question. He got this one right, but after he missed the next three, she switched gears.

"Finish what I say: After Kim broke the plate, Mother said, 'Don't cry over spilled _____.'" Holden didn't get many in this category correct unless Dr. Pratt prompted him twice or with the sound of the beginning of the word. Perhaps he hadn't heard some of these phrases before, but that was unlikely. He didn't even try to answer them.

In another part of the test, Dr. Pratt asked him to find absurdities. "What is silly about this picture?" The image depicted a man trying to read a newspaper while blindfolded.

"He's doing with a mask, white mask, yeah, trying to use a newspaper," Holden said.

"And this one? What is silly about this?" This image showed someone sweeping with an upside-down broom.

"That's a broom ... hmm ... broom-dust ... broom is missing ... upside down."

"Yes! Good job." *He's trying so hard to show us what he knows,* I thought.

Other tasks along these lines included a series of "What is missing from this picture?" questions. Dr. Pratt had asked two or three similar questions before moving to a different part of the test. Midway through the spiral-bound book, Holden struggled, fidgeting in his bed.

Dr. Pratt switched gears again, taking a chunky puzzle out of her bag and handing it to Holden. His eyes lit up, hands tickling the pieces as he turned them left and right to snap them into place in what seemed like record time.

"Thanks, Holden," Dr. Pratt said. "You did a great job." She didn't speak condescendingly to Holden. He gave her a meek smile, then turned to stare out the window.

* * *

Like the first test, he couldn't understand the questions—even more so this time. And the EEG revealed no changes. The first six months of medication failed to restore his language and failed to clear the seizure activity on the EEG. During Dr. Jones's brief consultation—the pediatric unit seemed busier than usual—he outlined his plan to tweak the medications. Dr. Pratt spent more time with me one-on-one to discuss other treatment possibilities. IVIG therapy was still a possibility, but the Minnesota Epilepsy Group (MEG) team considered it a last resort because the procedure took a toll on kids and didn't always work. Dr. Pratt then showed me a research article about multiple subpial transection (MST) and told me about her postdoctoral work with the surgeon in Chicago who performed the procedure. "The surgeon is very skilled, but it still doesn't always work," she said. She explained that Holden would come back to Children's to undergo sedation for a special kind of MRI so the neurosurgeon in Chicago could pinpoint where the seizures originated and how they spread. If the seizures occurred on both sides of his brain, which decreased the surgery's efficacy, Holden wouldn't be a candidate for MST.

When alone with Holden in his room, I opened my laptop and googled MST. Although a relatively new epilepsy treatment option, it seemed to be among the safest kinds of brain surgery. Performed via craniotomy, the surgeon cuts nerve fibres in the outer layer of the brain that pre-surgical imaging had deemed responsible for the seizure activity. The parallel transections are shallow cuts in the abnormal brain tissue and spare the parts of the brain responsible for vital functions found in the deeper layers. Imagining a surgeon opening up Holden's brain sent my heart into my stomach, but it also lit me up with excitement. As risky as I knew brain surgery could be, it could also mean a cure—a permanent clearing of the seizures that stole Holden's consciousness: they exhausted his body; they fogged his awareness; they limited the pleasures of the senses; they impeded his ability to communicate; they robbed him of memories; they jeopardized his life.

Since Holden was a child, it was my responsibility to make healthcare choices for him. I wanted to believe that MST would cure Holden, and I knew cures happened in other people's lives. Still, it felt dangerous to pin my hopes on a mere possibility. I wondered how long I'd have to wait to know whether Holden was a candidate or not.[10]

* * *

The only professional who spoke the word *disability* to me in the first year of the LKS diagnosis was the social worker employed by MEG, Lynn. During that hospital visit, when Lynn poked her head inside the door to Holden's room, I recalled that I'd met her before, but I didn't understand her job in relation to us. I was overwhelmed by the variety of professional designations among the staff: child life coordinators, who tried to make the hospital stays more pleasant; technicians, who oversaw the EEG leads and monitored the study; pediatric neurologists, medical doctors who specialized in children's brain issues; neuropsychologists, who had expertise in children's learning; and psychologists, who advised on behaviour. A social worker's role in the hospital context confused me.

"I think the last time I told you about family vouchers for food," Lynn said. She slid a chair closer to mine. She looked at me, searching my reaction, then proceeded to tell me about places in the hospital where families could get snacks and light meals at no cost. For a moment, I got lost in the directions but snapped back to attention when she asked whether I had health insurance for Holden.

"Holden has medical insurance through my work," I explained. "It's pretty good, but it doesn't cover everything. His dad and I split out-of-pocket expenses." My voice got quiet. Since the divorce, I'd managed expenses but couldn't save anything. Not having a cushion for emergencies made me nervous.

"Did you complete the Medicaid application I gave you during your last visit? Families often find Medicaid helpful—necessary even—with a disabled child."

"Um, no." Shame rose, my face flushing. I felt guilty for not completing this paperwork because if Holden qualified, it would provide some financial relief by covering the care my primary insurance wouldn't and by taking care of the copays and bills until I met my deductible. Something else besides guilt surfaced too. Discomfort. A profound discomfort I couldn't quite articulate. Lynn seemed to sense this and wrapped up her visit by explaining that I could complete the paperwork later, then left it near the door with her business card on top.

In a way, Lynn acted as my first disability doula. In *Care Work: Dreaming Disability Justice*, disability activist Leah Lakshmi Piepzna-Samarasinha interviews Stacey Milbern about their work to reconceptualize care that centres the agency of queer and disabled people of colour. Milbern and Piepzna-Samarasinha describe a disability doula as someone who helps rebirth someone as disabled or more disabled, which Milbern says could include "learning how to get medicine, drive a wheelchair, hire attendants, change a diet, date, have sex, make requests, code switch, live with an intellectual disability, go off meds, etc."[11] The need for a disability doula reveals practical changes one must make, and Lynn, by leaving the paperwork on the counter and saying the word *disability*, was the first to communicate, *You'll need help with this.*

Even though Lynn didn't exactly say that sentence, it hovered in my mind as my eyes flitted between the research article on MST and the stack of paper Lynn had left beside it. I read across them: regression, brain surgery, disability. Qualifying for Medicaid based on disability meant that this was a long-term issue. Medicaid wasn't for learning problems that could be addressed with tutoring or an occasional visit to a specialty clinic, and Lynn thought I would need it. She connected my role as Holden's mom to resources that would assist me and doing so made these elements visible. In *Care Work*, Milbern argues that the process of becoming disabled is often "invisibilized to the point that these changes do not even have a name."[12] I imagine that these relationships of care can also address the more philosophical, emotional, and attitudinal changes a person grapples with along the "spectrum of ability." This discussion, which I read nearly ten years after my interaction with Lynn, helped me identify Lynn's role in my life but also inspired me to imagine: What if someone could've given me some tips about meltdowns besides the advice that came from family and friends: *Just don't take Holden out*? What if someone could've pointed to experts on inclusion in schools? What if someone could've explained that there's a whole disability movement out there, and people have gone through this before?

Instead, as I sat in my discomfort mulling over Lynn's words, I felt myself reorienting from one reality to another, from one where a medical fix was likely (medication) to one where there would be no medical fix. Completing the application would mean confronting the fact that my son was disabled. And disabled felt like a label with weight. What did that mean for Holden? Not able to read? Not able to have a conversation with me? Not able to sustain friendships? Not able to be free of medications?

And did it mean that I would not be able, either? Not able to be free of constant vigilance? Not be released from this intense parenting? Not able to continue on this writer/teacher path I'd been walking for what felt like my whole life?

How could I both hold on to my dreams for my son—falling into books for hours, loving school, having friends over all the time, travelling with me, graduating from university, finding meaningful work, falling in love—and embrace this altered reality? How should I navigate my own dreams? I had no answers, and I didn't know to ask anyone else.

In *Care Work*, Piepzna-Samarasinha addresses the issue of asking for help in the context of disability: "What does it mean to wrestle with the ideas of softness and strength, vulnerability, pride, asking for help and not—all of which are deeply raced and classed and gendered?"[13] When I read this question the first time, nearly a decade after Holden was diagnosed with LKS, I cried. As a cisgender, nondisabled, financially secure white woman, I'm fairly certain I'm not the audience

Piepzna-Samarasinha imagined, but just the notion that one can ask for help felt emotionally destabilizing. I put down the book with guilt (why didn't I ask for help?), with shame (what does it say about my weakness as a mother that I didn't?), and with wonder (what would collaborative responsibility mean with a disabled child involved?). If I was the weaver of the Holden's care web, all I'd accomplished was one thread: a cohort of medical professionals a four-hour drive away. And because we paid them, I didn't even think they counted.

And yet my context—even as it meant some kinds of privilege—limited my ability to create a community of care for Holden. Piepzna-Samarasinha's experiences of collective care occurred in metropolitan cities with adults who could ask for and offer support to each other in the network. In Brookings—home to one grocery store, one Walmart, a few strip malls, and a quaint downtown—disability was most often invisible. The few disabled people that I knew lived with their families. Perhaps I could've departed from Piepzna-Samarasinha's reciprocity model and asked nondisabled friends, but my friendships felt fragile. Even before the LKS diagnosis, a few friends distanced themselves from our family: I saw eyebrows raise whenever they asked Holden a question that he didn't answer; I read judgment in their eyes whenever Holden had a meltdown; my kid was a brat, their body language seemed to say, and I was an indulgent parent. Even more fell away after Holden's care became more intense and Abel left. I didn't have time for spontaneous coffee dates and lunches, and after saying no a few times, I stopped getting invitations. Although I could talk to some friends about my experiences, few seemed to understand. I felt like an active friendship with me was a burden.

Perhaps the burden and shame I felt in asking for help is what made me double down on self-reliance. Instead of finding disability in lived realities, in communities comprised of disabled people, in movements for justice and using these lenses to reorient my life, I reacted by deciding what I would—what I could—do. I recalled how Holden resisted every single transition once we left the hotel and landed in the pediatric epilepsy unit. I recalled the blue burrito, how Holden's body eventually relaxed until tears streamed down his face. And then I went deeper into my memory, recalling IEP meetings, my research on LKS, Holden's outbursts—all the moments that could've helped me make the transition I'd been resisting, avoiding. It was time for me to submit to disability—even my partial understanding of it—before it became my blue burrito. Or perhaps my ignorance of it had been exactly that, and now I could be released.

* * *

Just before Dr. Jones sent the discharge orders, Dr. Pratt stopped by to see if I had any questions about MST. She asked Holden a question, and he responded with a one-word answer before his eyes looked away, his gaze resting on the window as if he was trying to find the source of a siren sounding outside the hospital. After a minute, his eyes turned back to us. "I think I'm losing my mind again," he said. That was the only complete and contextually appropriate sentence he'd uttered that day, perhaps in multiple days. I sat there, flabbergasted by the revelation that some part of him understood the impact of the seizures. I cried silently as Dr. Pratt slipped out of the room to give me some space to process this new layer of knowledge.

Chapter Eleven

INTERSTITIAL: a narrow opening

IN MAY 2013, BRIAN AND I WALKED INTO THE TATE GALLERY in London, a bit weary but recovered from jet lag. A banner for the exhibit *Poetry and Dream: Surrealism and Beyond* caught my attention.

"Look," I said, pointing it out. "It's as if I planned this visit just to see this!"

Brian was reading something on his phone. He pushed up his glasses, looked up and smiled an I'm-so-happy-that-you're-so-happy kind of grin, an our-love-still-feels-so-new kind of grin. Back in September, we'd hatched a plan: I'd apply for grant money to do research on Katherine of Aragon in London and Hildegard of Bingen in Germany, both writing interests of mine, and he'd lead a study-abroad trip for architecture students to both countries. We'd thrown the grant application together right before the deadline—the week after Holden's LKS diagnosis, when my mind was still reeling. I didn't think they'd award it.

But they did. And students signed up for Brian's trip. In March, we booked flights for the day after classes were over so we could get back before Holden's school year ended. I thought it would be easier to manage his care that way; he would stay with his dad for two weeks, and I arranged for a babysitter to help around the margins of Abel's workday. I hadn't expected that April EEG to add a layer of worry regarding regression and possible brain surgery. I hadn't expected that I'd begin to understand Holden's LKS as a permanent fixture in our lives.

"I think the students are already here somewhere," Brian said, looking around.

"Why don't you find them, go to the exhibits you want them to see, and we'll meet up later?" I squeezed his hand and went to find *Poetry and Dream.*

* * *

Ekphrasis comes from Greek: *ek*, meaning "out," and *phrazein*, meaning "to speak." And I find Elizabeth Loizeaux's definition of its rhetorical use apt: "a vivid description that would bring persons, places, things, ideas, and sometimes actions to the mind's eye of an audience."[1] I imagine ancient rhetors practising *ekphrasis* through exercises on description and precision—their words powerful enough to seal images in their audience's minds as they argued. Contemporary writers use it more loosely to describe written responses to visual works. Claire Barbetti emphasizes *ekphrasis* as a "contemplative act, a complex process of perception, memory, translation, interpretation and composition."[2] This definition describes my use, and working with the collection in the South Dakota Art Museum gave me ample practice engaging in its recursive process.[3]

Tourists and art lovers packed the Tate that day, and I wove among them looking for the west wing, level three. Walking through a place new to me sparked my attention, every sense cataloguing impressions. I was tuned into my observations when I found artists who explored dreams, the unconscious, and archetypal myth, beginning with Edward Wadsworth's *The Beached Margin*: stars and balls suspended from poles, bright red against blue sky and golden sand. Next I paused before Man Ray's *Pisces 1938*—the female nude stretched parallel to a mackerel. As I catalogued textures and shapes and colour, I felt my shoulders relax—the beginning of ekphrastic perception. I connected information from the art descriptions with my own observations. Whether they perplexed me or compelled analysis, poems were born.

My favourite surrealist pieces featured words-as-image; embedded words among geometric elements generated questions. Roland Penrose's *Portrait* included painted lines: "his thighs windmills" and "arms canary cages." I wondered why he used words instead of images. On others' paintings I wondered if words were simply shapes or if the meaning of the word itself held importance. I smiled despite myself. Before learning a bit about how to interpret artwork—largely through conversations with Brian—I wouldn't have had these questions. We often discussed the ways words worked as elements as well as the ways meanings morphed across context and time. He'd poked fun at my use of Times New Roman typeface and wondered why I didn't care about how my words looked on a page. Much as I had viewed surrealistic art in the past, I had no idea what he was talking about. Weren't the words' meanings all that mattered? No. He chose a specific font for composition because it altered the way he thought about the content. These sorts of conversations were always popping up—me schooling him in the ways creative nonfiction could be creative, him breaking open new ways of seeing design. As we discussed our work and our parallel artistic processes, we built layers of intellectual intimacy.

I moved into the "Realisms" section of the exhibit, pausing longest in front of Dod Procter's *Morning* (1926). The sleeping woman—her thick legs sticking out of sheets, full hips wrapped in a bedsheet the same colour as her nightshirt—made me catch my breath. *That's me,* I thought, although the woman didn't really look like me in the face. Nor was I as youthful. And yet she slept on her left side, right leg on top of left, torso twisted at the waist—my habit too. The bed, clothes, and sheet were variations of white-grey; her skin, washed out by the morning light, seemed iridescent. In this image, I saw my profound yearning for rest realized.

At home, Holden slept alongside me most nights. He'd fall asleep in his own bed, settled by books and a hug, but he'd wake up after midnight. Sometimes, he'd wander down the hall to crawl in bed next to me. He tossed and turned, rolling away with the covers and kicking me with his foot. Sometimes, if he had full-blown insomnia, he'd play in his room loud enough to wake me up, and I'd try to coax him back to sleep. He rarely did, so we'd watch a movie, dozing on the couch. On the nights he slept well, I didn't. I'd wake up on my own, perhaps from an unremembered nightmare, unable to settle down until I studied his blankets for the up-and-down of his breath. The nights when I'd sleep for eight hours and wake up well-rested seemed as if they'd happened in another life.

On the trip, anxiety gripped me when I thought about Holden. A deep breath usually stemmed the panic. It was day four in London, and each morning I'd woken up worried. As soon as Brian left on a breakfast run, I'd check my email for news about Holden from Abel and from Holden's teacher, so I'd be assured by the time he came back with coffee and pastries. *You can't alter every aspect of your life because of Holden's epilepsy,* I'd think. Then I'd counter it with, *Well, you already have; you owe yourself this break, this trip.* I toggled back and forth between feeling self-indulgent and feeling proud of myself for trusting Holden's care to his father, sitter, and teachers. This back-and-forth kept worry at the ready. One afternoon, I snapped a photo of the Paddington Bear statue in Paddington Station because it would amuse Holden, but then I just kept thinking of Holden's sweet face and in seconds, a wave of nausea swept through me. *What if he needed me and I wasn't there?* I calculated the hours between us, and I called Abel, praying he'd pick up. He reported that Holden was fine. Every time my heart lurched, I'd remind myself his dad could handle an emergency. And I needed to travel and work so I could remain a healthy mother. After a few minutes, calmness resumed.

In the Tate, the anxiety had begun to wane when I walked up to Meredith Frampton's *Marguerite Kelsey* (1928). Uncorseted yet slender in a cream-coloured dress, the sitter was beautiful: parted brown hair pulled back at the nape, muted makeup on her high cheekbones, slender nose, heavy-lidded eyes. Everything about the composition felt crafted: sage drape, brown wall, black chaise, magnolia bouquet. Her red shoes struck me. *I'd wear those in a hot minute,* I thought. And her gaze? Discerning. Determined. I saw myself in that gaze.

Before layering ekphrasis into my writing practice, I wasn't used to seeing anything about myself reflected in art—not the way I slept, and certainly not the expression on someone's face. But the contemplative act of reading art aligned with the contemplative process of writing, and I found myself expanding into the images. Studying *Marguerite Kelsey*, I imagined that a discerning, determined look was my expression on my best days. Since the LKS diagnosis, moments of wanting to disappear no longer happened—perhaps because the diagnosis gave me a place to start piecing a way forward, perhaps because my relationship with Brian made me feel more alive. Probably both. I wanted to be a good mother to Holden and protect what made me *me* before he was born, which meant doing what I needed to do as a woman, as a writer. Those red shoes. The trip to London.

By the time I found the handful of Picasso paintings in the exhibit, Brian had caught up. "What do you think?" he asked, standing next to me. I took his arm by the elbow.

"I didn't think I liked Picasso, based on what I've seen in books, but I love this one. It's so sensual," I said. *Nude Woman in a Red Armchair* (1932) seemed a series of curves: curved chair holding curvy hips anchoring curvy breasts.

"Do you see how it's doubled? Her face is split in two—mirrored in a way—but the blue part could be her lover," Brian said. I turned my head to the side and saw it. The doubled-ness made me re-see her eyes—not wistful but reflective.

"It evokes the possibility of pleasure," I replied.

Brian nodded. I slipped my hand into his and caught his scent, a mix of patchouli, hair gel, and *him*. My heartbeat quickened. His fingers curving around mine sparked memories of all the places they'd touched me.

As we held hands and looked at the portrait in silence, the pleasures I took from the Picasso and the rush of desire I felt for Brian amused me. My sense of art was certainly changing, I thought. Was my sense of myself changing too? Perhaps. Or perhaps I was simply reawakening the parts of me muted by stress and sleeplessness, by anxiety and change.

I grasped Brian's hand, and he turned to me with a full-of-love smile. We kissed right there in front of the Picasso, then turned away in a giddy silence to look for Brian's students on a different floor.

* * *

Brian left London a few days before I did to visit a Czech university that offered a study-abroad semester program for his students. His absence gave me time alone with a research interest: Katherine of Aragon. Katherine, Henry VIII's first wife, intrigued me because Henry divorced her after she had one child and a number of miscarriages. As I walked in the kitchens of Hampton Court Palace, I focused my perception, taking in details of walls and stone hearths. I remembered from my reading that Katherine had spent time in the kitchens, so I imagined her walking nearby to supervise the massive work needed to sustain the palace. In the long corridors, I imagined her hating the cold, dank weather, and longing for her childhood home in Spain. As I walked outside, I wondered if she had stood there, too, reflecting on her lost pregnancies. In the chapel—perhaps the only room changed little from Katherine's time—I recalled the strength her Catholic faith gave her to fight the humiliation of Henry's divorce. I became wistful for the time when religion strengthened me, too.

At the palace, I took photos that inspired poems: carved pomegranates in the Great Hall, chapel drapery, gardens. Mine were visceral, imagistic impressions that I translated later in compositions. I took deep breaths and imagined us looking at the river from the same angle but in different centuries. I couldn't fathom what it meant to be royalty or what it meant to live in Renaissance England, but I knew what it felt like to hear the word "divorce." I knew what it meant to survive miscarriages and secondary infertility. I knew what it meant to love an only child.[4]

Between visits to historic places and museums, I wrote for hours in coffee shops. My iPad and discerning eye transformed the objects and scenes into photographs—some more artful than others. In a book about the pedagogical uses of *ekphrasis*, Terry Blackhawk writes that "Art requires leaps of perceiving and experiencing," and that art encounters can "provide poets with an imaginative substratum through which difficult personal subjects can surface."[5] I studied snapshots of portraits and pomegranates and Paddington Bears, leaping through the images of these objects into the emotional impressions they conjured. Katherine of Aragon's pomegranates became grenades and watchful, explosive eyes; hallways of the laundry inspired letters to the late queen. I imagined whole scenes between Katherine and Henry, and I revisited the parallel scenes between me and my ex-husband.

When I settled into writing, anxiety evaporated. Time dissolved into words. Even though sorrow and stress surfaced in the subjects, the process gave me distance. The practice of ekphrasis felt like both buffer and balm. I wondered whether the process of parenting Holden would ever feel so familiar to me as writing did—so oddly comforting even as it challenged and demanded and provoked me. I hoped it would.

* * *

As a process, *ekphrasis* is relational: I relate artwork to my experience or to story or to another piece of art. Monica Prendergast defines *ekphrastic* inquiry in precisely this way, as "a way of understanding one kind of experience in terms of another."[6] But it's not a one-to-one correspondence that reduces possibility; because the "terms of another" are in a different medium, the *ekphrastic* process introduces additional elements: shape, texture, colour, composition, etc. By suggesting fresh interpretations and opening up other ways of seeing, I'm compelled to think in new ways. Sometimes, the practice of thinking through the artwork encourages me to make new meaning or revise my sense of an experience I thought I understood. This cultivates a relationship to the imaginary where possible futures develop.

Diagnostic frames can serve to narrow; ekphrastic frames can serve to expand because they resist rigidity and invite imagination. After summoning memory and offering associations, ekphrastic frames can become points of departure for new art. Sometimes frames are pages; sometimes canvases. By the time I landed in Berlin, the sensory immersion of travel and ekphrastic inquiry of my work made me default to framing. I engaged everything as art.

Arriving in Berlin felt dreamy. I gave the German cabdriver directions to the address Brian had supplied, but I barely kept my eyes open to make sure he followed them. I was relieved when we pulled over somewhere in the city and Brian appeared, paid the driver, and grabbed my bag.

"I missed you," he said, hugging me. We kissed in the middle of the sidewalk, the flow of pedestrians shifting for our embrace.

"It was only three days," I said. But I'd missed him too. "How was Prague?" I looked around as he swung my bag over his shoulder, expecting to see a hotel among the tall buildings. Nothing looked familiar. I followed Brian down the narrow sidewalk, chatting with him about what I'd seen without him, when suddenly he ducked inside the door of a concrete, Communist-era building. "We're staying here?" I asked as we lugged my bags past a wall of steel mailboxes and random flyers taped to peeling paint. "This place seems strange."

"Trust me," he said. "Wait until morning." After a long elevator ride, we stepped into a studio apartment: living/sleeping space, kitchenette, bathroom. I threw my backpack on the floor, used the bathroom, and melted into sleep.

Hours later, I woke with a start. Remembering what Brian had said, I stumbled over our bags and nearly tripped over a chair leg, but then my hand landed on the wall-length curtain thick enough to eclipse the sunrise. It was the only window in the place. I pulled it open and gasped.

We were twenty-three floors up. I felt in the sky myself, the hazy grey softening to blue just beyond the glass, just beyond me. I was in the frame. And below? Layers: the horizon of city, buildings and parks, Alexanderplatz, a maze of streets, the *Hackescher Markt* train station. How long did I stand there watching the city wake up? Trains sighed and cars beeped, sounds drifting up to the dizzying height.

A catalogue of snapshot memories opened, previous moments of great height and great excitement when my body tuned to an intense emotional frequency: the view from the Eiffel Tower, the landscape at Mt. Washington, the city below the Space Needle, the glittering thread of the Euphrates from Mt. Nemrut. Each time, I'd felt this thrill—the thrill of stepping into the frame, the thrill of *being* the subject, not the maker.

What would it mean to relate living to art? That is, to understand living not as following the single-track Plan but as composing a series of artworks? To use the recursive processes of drafting and revision to move in and out of frames or margins, to be both subject and maker? It would mean a need to sharpen my discernment, living in smaller chunks of time, valuing the messy, understanding the process as the stable element, not the product.

I recalled the last few months with Holden, and I recognized how the intensity of parenting felt similar to the process of composing poems: I sank time and effort into the work without knowing what the outcome would be. Of course, there's far less at stake when writing poems compared to raising a child, but thinking through parenting by thinking through art felt capacious and filled with possibility—emotions that The Plan never afforded me. Suddenly, I wanted to remember every detail of this moment of standing in the frame. I tried to soak in the city, my eyes acting like hands to touch the textures of buildings, to feel the heat of concrete, to apprehend the city's vibrations.

The morning's sunshine honeyed everything—the trains, the buildings, my hands on the glass—with a glow. I wouldn't get this exact kind of moment again, but that didn't mean I wouldn't experience it in a different context. I'd have to revise my life and use the ever-unfolding process of composing to help. I glanced behind me at Brian, who still slept. Wasn't our relationship evidence of revision? I turned back to the city, and even though my heart pumped as hard and fast as I'd ever remembered it, I pressed my forehead and toes against the glass. Tingling from my hands and feet spread to my entire body. It seemed as if the heat I generated could dissolve the entire window.

When I finally stepped down, I began to sense a change; I began to trust my process of living just as I trusted my process of writing.

* * *

Berlin was magical in the same way Brian was intense: always moving, creating, revealing something new. Before that trip, our dates in coffee shops, kitchens, and beds were bookended by responsibilities: Holden to feed, classes to hold, meetings to attend. In Europe, we'd never woken up together so many mornings in a row or shared so many consecutive meals. I learned that he could skip breakfast and lunch (not ideal, but possible), and that he preferred espresso once a day at any time of day. And his intensity wasn't confined to just a few hours; every waking moment he listened and read and absorbed information through music and film and text. He fought off pain after a day of walking with his artificial knee—the result of a cancerous tumour he'd had removed in his early thirties—and he fought through a twenty-four-hour flu. And when I proposed renting a car to facilitate my research on Hildegard, I fell asleep to him studying Autobahn road maps in German.

Brian was at his most intense in Berlin, a place he'd once lived. Every corner had a story—historical, architectural, personal. In Berlin, I discovered the wonder of seeing a city via bicycle (biking was also easier on Brian's knee.) I also discerned the architectural magic of the *Neue Nationalgalerie*, Altes Museum, *Berliner Dom*, and *Staatsbibliothek.* We toured churches made from rammed earth, visited the Berggruen Museum, and walked in silence at the Memorial to the Murdered Jews of Europe. Brian told stories he'd learned about the Second World War, the divided city, and the wall's fall, about who built what and why. Every moment in Berlin held the promise of learning—always the spark of composition.

The day we parked our bikes outside the courtyard of the *Nationalgalerie Hamburger Bahnhof,* he wore his cherry-red pants, bright blue Converse, and an even brighter blue T-shirt. He made it easy for me to follow him in traffic. We were both tired, but Andy Warhol's *Ten-Foot Flowers* next to his *Camouflage* energized me. The latter reminded me of a coveted blanket that my father brought back from his military service in Vietnam, the one my brother and I had fought over to build forts in our living room; I was probably reading behind that blanket when Warhol was painting the light-infused greens. Roy Lichtenstein's work didn't prompt any memories, but I appreciated the stacked geometries of *Imperfect Painting* and its contrasts of yellow, maroon, and mauve. I wondered how the artists made the art—the material elements and the physical work of production—making a mental note to do some follow-up research. But the only set of works that made lasting impact on me was *secret universe.*

"What do you think of these?" I asked Brian, pointing to one of George Widener's mixed-media-on-paper pieces. The blue background appeared dyed with indigo. A river of canary-yellow ovals flowed down the centre, some two or three abreast, each oval outlined in red with a date stamped on it in black. The other pieces, too, were arrangements of dates on a page. One portrayed black circles gathered in a massive oval on grey paper, numbers assigned to each circle.

"Why the dates?" Brian asked.

We read the description on the wall, which explained that Widener was autistic and that he had developed a preference for numbers, numerology, calendars, historical data, population statistics, and mathematical computations. Brian studied the piece a bit longer. I continued to read from the description: "When he looks at numbers or works on calculations, automatically images emerge in front of his inner eye. His brain automatically links different information levels, giving him access to worlds of perception that remain sealed to us."

Brian raised an eyebrow. "They're interesting," he said. He continued to study them, even though I knew the suggestion of hard-wired perceptual differences made him skeptical. That's exactly what intrigued me, though. Holden hadn't been diagnosed as autistic, but his brain worked visually. Deeper into the biographical information on Widener, I read that he dropped out of an engineering program, but later went to a university that featured a program for people with disabilities. He credited this liberal-arts education with helping him figure out how to live a more balanced life and how to be a successful artist.

"Sometimes you just never know how someone will use their differences creatively," I said as we walked out of the gallery. Perhaps I should enroll Holden in some art classes when I get home, I thought. Perhaps there will be possibilities for Holden I can't even imagine now.

* * *

In my relationship with Brian, there have been many occasions when I understand that we are consciously composing together, where we move in and out of *responding* to experience, sometimes even stepping into the frame. Perhaps it's because he, too, composes his life in similar ways, although he'd use different words to describe that approach. Our decision to get married felt like one of those co-created moments.

Two months after returning from Europe, toward the end of July, I headed to Cottonwood Café to write for an hour. I'd been asked to give a poetry keynote address in early October, so I'd begun to prepare.

That morning, I was writing a multilayered poem inspired by the illustration *Women Collecting Cocoons and Weaving Silk* from an illuminated manuscript.[7] I sipped my cappuccino as I brainstormed the way moving from one house to another felt like the transformation of caterpillar to butterfly—a reduction to stem cells and complete rebuilding of a body. A text from Brian interrupted: Meet me at Cottonwood?

A few minutes later, I watched through the glass as Brian rolled up on his bike. He wore a short-sleeved button-down shirt and shorts, which meant he had plans to make something in the shop with his students and probably didn't have any meetings scheduled. He moved his messenger bag off his shoulder and walked in.

"Do you need anything?" He sat down. Then he got back up again.

"No, thanks. I have my coffee already."

He looked at it, then me.

"Do you have the poem with you?" he asked. "The one you read at the reading here?"

"Yes, I think so. Why?" He'd never asked me for a poem out of the blue.

"Can you find it?" He looked over his shoulder as he walked to the counter.

"Sure," I said. I pulled up "All My Engineering" and emailed it to him, thinking he wanted a copy of it for something. A few minutes later he sat down, latte in hand.

"I emailed you the poem."

"Oh. I wanted you to read it."

"Like, read it to you? Right ... now?"

"Would you?"

"Sure." I opened the document again, feeling my eyebrows knit together. "I want to engineer / us, so I sketch black lines..." I read through the Frank Lloyd Wright reference, and stopped after the next line: "Structures quicken my heart." I glanced up. He was looking at me, eyes watery. He took out a brown gift bag from his messenger bag.

The week before, we'd gone for a long bike ride, as we often did when Holden was with his dad—and we talked intensely the whole way. We discussed raising Holden; Brian described how he liked his role as an extra in Holden's life (his dad living close by), and I explained my worries about seizures and LKS. We talked about our jobs; he admired my writing and loved that we were both professors, and I admired how he was building a department and loved the way he talked about teaching. We talked about our past marriages, and we named our fears. At the end of the bike ride, we'd reached a new level of understanding. At the end of the bike ride, I knew what I'd say if he ever asked.

I returned to the poem:

> If only 'relationship building'
> meant five-hour What If sessions
> surfing possibilities, library
> books spilling out of my bag,
> magazines coffee-stained, your
> shadow over me at the keyboard.

I saw our current life in the poem—a poem I'd begun months before we started dating.

> It's the stories we'll write
> with that bedroom, this bathroom

I rushed through the next lines and looked up at the end. Brian pushed the gift bag toward me. Inside, a tiny box. I popped it open, revealing an oval sapphire ring with four diamonds on each side secured with a white-gold band. I raised my eyes to meet his. Without his glasses in the way, his hazel eyes were unobstructed. He nodded slightly.

"It's beautiful!" I pulled it out of the box. And then I stumbled, unsure of where to put the ring. "Um ... do you have any words to go with this?"

He did. And I said yes to them all.

Chapter Twelve

INTERNALIZE: to incorporate within oneself

IN ALISON KAFER'S *Feminist, Queer, Crip*, SHE ARGUES AGAINST the *curative imaginary*: "an understanding of disability that not only *expects* and *assumes* intervention but also cannot imagine or comprehend anything other than intervention."[1] This way of thinking, often the default/dominant paradigm, was my framework for understanding Holden's seizure disorder at the beginning: What medication would stop the seizures? What treatment would bring his language back? What could I expect in terms of progress? Perhaps because my early encounters framed a seizure disorder from a medical perspective, or because of my fear that Holden would die, I imagined cure as seizure-free, with language resumed and behaviour normalized. Kafer states that in the curative imaginary, "the only appropriate disabled mind/body" submits to treatments to eliminate impairments and assimilate into normalcy.[2] The curative imaginary enforces linearity—a movement out of disability that accretes and re-forms—and reduces success to progress. From the first diagnosis of epilepsy to well into the first year after the

LKS diagnosis, I unwittingly employed a curative imaginary. And yet, despite not knowing the better frames that Kafer uses to think about disabled futures, I'd begun to "do the present differently" that summer after returning from Europe.

The night I returned from Berlin and two full months before Brian's proposal of marriage, I dozed watching a movie with Holden. Exhausted from travel and jet lag, I sank into a deep sleep. The slam of the front door startled me awake. Holden, who had been curled up against me in his blanket, was gone. I stumbled to the front door calling his name; I thought I would find him playing on the steps or driveway, but no.

I panicked. Where could he have run so quickly? The neighbours' yards to the north of the street were empty. He wasn't running out of the cul-de-sac in that direction at least, I thought. I walked to the end of our yard and looked south—and there he was, strolling under the streetlights three houses away. He wouldn't turn around or come back when I called his name. A few days later, he left out the front door while I was in the bathroom; I found him in my neighbour's car, the same model and colour as mine. Another time he was inspecting a motorcycle in a neighbour's open garage. Holden didn't seem able to think through danger as he once did, and he couldn't communicate the reasons for his actions, if there were any.

I started to imagine him slipping out of the house more often without me knowing. I saw him lost in a field a few streets down. I pictured him hit by a car on Main Avenue. I pictured a stranger pull him into a van from the sidewalk. I pictured a police car slow down, and when the officer tried to engage Holden, I saw Holden run. What, then, would the officer do? A new strand of anxiety began to weave its way through the fabric of my life.

But at the same time, a shift had begun. No longer tied to The Plan, agency surfaced; I felt open to change. If I couldn't keep Holden safe in this house, I should find another. What had once seemed impossible to consider seemed the best solution: selling my house.

On real estate websites, I looked for something safer and easier to maintain. *Simplify,* I thought. *You don't have time for a garden anymore.* I could only accomplish outside chores when Holden was at daycare because I couldn't leave him alone in the house to work outside, and if I took him outside with me, he often slipped out one of three gates. When we were inside, he couldn't play in the walk-out basement by himself; even if I alarmed all the doors, it would take me a minute or two to track him down if one went off. Plus, I was struggling to keep the house clean while also grocery shopping and cooking and working full-time.

I kept returning to photos of a condo close to campus. Reasonably priced, it featured a private, plant-filled courtyard. It had three doors: one to the garage, which would have the extra barrier of the garage door; one to the courtyard, which was accessible but less so if padlocked, and a front door, which could be monitored fairly easily. All plusses. Minuses? Outdated and half the space of my house. *Create a life to reflect your reality,* I thought, *not the dreams you had when you moved to Brookings.* The reasons I'd chosen my house—big yard, space for two children, an open-concept area good for entertaining—no longer fit.

In the middle of June, Brian and I looked at the condo together and went out for coffee afterward. I asked him what he, as a professor of architecture, thought of the place. His response surprised me: "When I moved here, that condo complex was the only place I considered living in besides the apartment I ended up renting. I haven't owned a house before, but I like it."

As we discussed its pros and cons, he sketched the condo out on a napkin. Delighted, I blurted out, "Well, would you want to live there too?" Then I tacked on, "You know, someday." Perhaps this had been my proposal moment—a full six weeks before his. He looked at me and smiled. "Yes. Yes, I would."

* * *

By the second week of July, after securing the condo, I cleared my schedule as much as possible to enact *sell-house-fast mode*. But my house needed a lot of work, and prepping it disrupted my sense of time. In order to move forward physically, I had to move backwards emotionally. For two weeks, plus four more weeks of partial days, I sorted, packed, and repaired. When a space was cleared, I prettied it up: new carpet for the basement, new shelves, and new mirrors for the bathrooms. Every repair and pruned shrub reflected a reason, a meaning, a memory. Packing and sorting felt like confrontation.[3]

In the closet-sized bathroom where I had miscarried pregnancies, I sorted lotion, makeup, and nail polish into boxes and stowed them away. I pried off the mirror and rust-spotted medicine cabinet. I took paint to be stirred and masked the edges of the countertops. Then I watched fresh paint eclipse the washed-out walls I'd stared at as I bled.

New paint. New walls. It seemed so easy—a bit of time, effort, elbow grease. But it felt like breaking concrete to remake that room and renegotiate the memories it held.

In Holden's room, I knelt in front of his shelves: on my left, a pile of boxes for books to move to the condo; on my right, a pile of plastic bags for books to give away. I touched the spines of books from his babyhood: *Winnie-the-Pooh's Opposites*; *First 100 Words*; *Goodnight, Moon*; *My Many Colored Days*; *My First Dinosaur: Touch and Feel*. *My Many Colored Days* fell off the shelf, its cardboard frayed at the ends. I opened to a page with a red horse, smudged as if painted by a child: "On Bright Red Days / how good it feels / to be a horse / and kick my heels!" Holden loved naming the feelings of the day. Brown days were sad, purple days lonely, yellow days busy. *He couldn't even name his feelings anymore,* I thought. *And he is already too old for this book.* I realized I'd been keeping it for the sibling he was supposed to have. I tossed it into the plastic donation bag, then waffled. It would be a great book for his keepsake box, but would he value keepsakes? I hoped he would, so I took it out and put it into a box, scribbling "Keepsakes" on the side. Those for more advanced reading I decided to keep. *Be optimistic,* I thought. *He'd learn to read eventually, right?*

His toys were harder to assess. I started with board games, holding *Orchard* in my hands. I remembered teaching him how to set up the cherries, pears, and plums on the trees; we had to harvest the fruit before the raven ate everything. He loved it. But he couldn't remember the rules anymore; he couldn't remember to take turns. I kept it anyway. Others, like *Chutes and Ladders* and *Candyland*, I donated. For each kind of toy—games, cars, or superheroes—I asked: Were there too many rules? Would Holden ever play with it? If the seizures subsided, would he be too old for the toy? Every few minutes, a toy would conjure a happy memory, and I'd tear up, then plow ahead. Sometimes, I considered myself delusional to hope that he'd someday play again; I'd already packed away his LEGO because, even though it didn't require language or rules, he'd started putting bricks into his mouth.

Packing Holden's room illuminated the strain and consequences of trying to imagine his future. His joy of game-playing seemed lost, which made me sad, and yet I didn't insist on a cure or believe he would remain the same. It seems I was thinking of Holden as "out of sync." Alongside the curative imaginary, Kafer explains how time can be rendered queer by disability, how illness can create strange temporalities where linear time becomes "out of joint": "The strange temporality of diagnosis/prognosis seems all the more dislocating, all the more dis- and reorienting, for those falling out of diagnostic categories."[4] Holden had a diagnosis, but there was no prognosis; he could make progress again, then regress—a cycle I was beginning to apprehend. And still, Dr. Jones told me that these seizures would end someday—not knowing exactly when, how, or to what extent felt dislocating. I didn't understand that strange temporalities could replace the curative imaginary's implied timeline, yet I was experiencing it.

I pushed myself to stretch, to shift, to work out of sync with the house—the place of old dreams, unusable timelines. When thoughts of failure crept in (my inability to care for the house and yard, yes, but also the miscarriages and failed marriage), I tried to talk myself into a good space: acknowledging my faults and letting go. And I didn't have to reorient alone. When Brian returned from a two-week trip to Canada, he excavated the storage space in the garage and the workroom in the basement, jettisoning wood and carpentry supplies stored there by previous owners. Together, we sold big items the condo couldn't contain (treadmill, bookcases, tables) and moved boxes from my house into the condo's garage. Right before we dubbed my house market-ready, I hired a contractor for the condo renovation that Brian designed.

Undoing my garden felt the most crushing. I undid the herb spiral section, pulling up dill, cilantro, and oregano by the stems. The roots blanched under the sun. I hauled cement pavers, one by one, from the heart of my yard and set them beside my front step. I freecycled them, imagining someone using them for a patio or playhouse. Then I disassembled my compost area with a pitchfork, displacing a garter snake, its slim-ribbon body disappearing into the grass. I filled wheelbarrow after wheelbarrow with compost, piles glittering with grubs and fat worms. My neighbours received three years' worth of saving and turning. Finally, I yanked out the yawning bloom of a volunteer squash.

Moving made me shift full circle—from seeding, nurturing, inventing, conceiving, to tearing down, removing, ruining. To clear a space for starting over made destruction an act of trust—trusting that change would ensue even when the details of that change remained unknown.

* * *

Kafer argues that in the curative imaginary, disability "must always be accompanied by a nostalgia for the lost able mind/body." That nostalgia prompts questions familiar to most disabled people: "Wouldn't you rather be cured? Wouldn't you like to be as you were before?"[5] Before the trip to Europe, before the move, before making a commitment to Brian about our future, nostalgia informed my emotional stance on being Holden's mom. I'd wanted Holden as he was before, since that meant, in my mind, safety and the comfort of The Plan. Yet that summer, doing the present differently enabled me to take a different stance. I began to work to access resources and therapies for Holden that would support him in the present—not some imagined future or some golden past. Between packing and cleaning, I translated the research I'd done post-diagnosis into action.

One support included obtaining American Sign Language (ASL) education for Holden, as well as lessons for myself. At Holden's April neuropsychological appointment with Dr. Pratt, I mentioned the research I'd found about using ASL to teach children with LKS. Because ASL—complete with its own grammar—developed independently of auditory processing, the language was understood using a different part of the brain than those affected by Holden's seizures.[6] In a discussion group I'd found on social media, another parent wrote that immersing her son in a school for the Deaf had made all the difference for academic progress once his seizures subsided. I resisted the possibility of future progress and instead reasoned that if Holden could learn a different form of communication now, it could ease his frustration and provide another avenue for self-expression. Dr. Pratt had read the research too and recommended ASL for Holden in her report. At his IEP meeting, the special education team agreed not only to hire a Deaf educator for Holden in second grade but also to help me find ASL classes.

That summer, I drove down to Sioux Falls once a week to learn basic grammar and vocabulary at the South Dakota Association of the Deaf. Teachers and parents of Deaf and hard-of-hearing children, including Holden's dad, comprised the group of twelve in ASL 1. The engaging instructor was enthusiastic about helping Holden. He shared a newspaper article about teaching ASL to a nonspeaking autistic teen and was open to teaching ASL to hearing folks who needed alternative forms of communication.

I also advocated for Holden's education in ASL. The district's special education director agreed that Holden needed to learn to sign but had concerns. "It's not enough to just find someone who uses or interprets ASL. It needs to be someone trained in teaching ASL and academics," she said. "That will be tough to find." I read this as a possible "I'm appearing supportive because I know this won't work out" move, which I'd witnessed administrative types employ before. But she did have a point: Brookings was a college town in a rural context. So I helped the director by contacting the program coordinators at all the regional schools that credentialed teachers in Deaf education to see if they knew of any students looking for jobs. Through those phone conversations, I learned about places to advertise the position beyond the usual district website, and one of those websites was how Holden's second-grade teacher found the job.

I secretly hoped that both Holden and I would become so proficient in ASL that we could carry on a conversation together—evidence of the curative imaginary's hold. Although neither of us ever gained a significant vocabulary, our developing knowledge often helped prevent and deescalate meltdowns. By the six-month mark, Holden could sign a dozen or so words, and when I signed, ASL helped him understand.

For example, I spoke *which* when I showed him a bagel and a box of cereal, but I also signed it—thumbs up, fingers tucked, moving back and forth. *Wait*—palms open, fingers moving up and down—was another I signed often. Holden signed *yes* and *no* the most often.

Another support I pursued was music therapy. I'd read that music therapy helped people with aphasia because the brain processes music and language in different parts. Like ASL, I hoped it would provide him a venue for self-expression. Once a week, we drove to Sioux Falls, where a music therapist worked with Holden in her basement-turned-studio. At the first lesson, Holden was scared and a bit overwhelmed by all the percussion instruments and guitars that filled the room. When he relaxed, he started singing—a song about counting animals.

The fluctuating nature of LKS meant that on some days Holden engaged with his teacher, but on others, not so much. Sometimes he wanted to play instruments roughly or in a different order; sometimes he didn't want to sing and refused any kind of participation. I couldn't cancel and reschedule on the bad days; the teacher's policy wasn't flexible. And the price—which I paid out of pocket since it wasn't covered by insurance—was steep. At first, the teacher tried to be patient and optimistic, but after a few weeks, I could tell that she didn't look forward to working with him. She didn't understand how seizure activity shaped Holden's behaviour, nor how insomnia and medication affected his abilities to attend to tasks and participate. Like all the other teachers, she analyzed his behaviour as if he could make choices like other kids. By mid-autumn, Holden's meltdowns and the teacher's pessimism made the effort seem less worth the drive and the price tag.

Perhaps the biggest support I sought for Holden was a service dog. I'd stumbled upon an article about how service dogs can be trained for autistic kids; they become loyal companions, help soothe meltdowns, and facilitate relationships. Around that same time, I'd watched a NOVA television special about how dogs can read human emotions and vice versa, which reinforced my beliefs about the power of human–canine relationships. But finding trainers in South Dakota proved impossible, and a group of trainers in North Dakota turned down our application because Holden wasn't old enough to take some responsibility for the dog. So I left a message at Pawsitivity in Minnesota, who trained dogs for kids in particular. I heard back toward the end of summer. Tom, one of the two-member team, told me that they'd started training a fifty-pound golden retriever, Haven, and invited me to apply to their program. Two days later, he called with the news: Holden was a match for Haven.

Holden and Haven met for the first time that September. On the four-hour drive to St. Paul, I wondered how it would go. The first few weeks of second grade had been rocky, even with a great new teacher. I tried to shrug off fretting as we got out of the car at our meeting spot, a park-like space in a posh part of the city. I hoped that meeting Haven would mark the beginning of something amazing for Holden, but I'd been wrong before.

"You must be Holden." Tom grinned as the two of us approached. Holden and I looked at Tom—his fashionable jeans, pointed shoes, and corduroy jacket—for only a second before Haven absorbed our attention. She sat alert but still. "You can pet her," Tom said. Holden put his right hand on top of her head and stroked her back, bending over to make sure he petted her all the way to her tail. "Strangers can't pet her unless they ask you and you say yes. Unlike other service dogs, she can be a social bridge." Holden stood up, and Tom and I continued our introductions as we followed the sidewalk to an open space beside a building.

Haven seemed curious about us but didn't tug on the leash. Holden walked behind me in silence. In the side yard, Tom unclipped Haven, pulled a tennis ball out of his bag, and threw it for her. She chased it across a thin stretch of lawn surrounded by hedge. Holden's eyes followed with excitement.

"Why don't you throw the ball for her, Holden?" Tom said. We chatted for a couple of minutes until Holden's interest in playing fetch with Haven waned. I was in the middle of a sentence when Holden bolted, running toward the hedge. Haven followed. I panicked, worried that they'd both run through the hedge and into traffic.

"Haven!" Tom called. She came back on the third call. I intercepted Holden with plenty of time. Crisis averted, I imagined.

For another hour, Tom and I discussed the responsibility of a service dog and the ways Haven could help Holden. Holden played with his iPad and Haven sat nearby. Tom explained that a primary bond between Holden and Haven would—at least theoretically—prompt her to alert me if Holden was having a seizure or otherwise seemed to need help. I hoped the seizure-alert function wouldn't be tested, but it also bolstered my sense of safety.

"Haven will have a lot of responsibility," I said, looking at her sweet face.

"Officially, yes, and she'll have a lot of unofficial jobs, too," Tom said. He listed cuddling and being cute among them.

We also discussed walking, feeding, and reinforcing Haven's training—all things Tom said he'd remind me about when her training was complete. Some tips I already knew, since my family had always had dogs, but I appreciated them, having never owned one myself.

"She likes going for walks, but Haven really enjoys just hanging out, too," Tom said.

Hearing her name, Haven put her face on Holden's leg, and I fell completely in love with the idea of Haven and Holden. *She's so loving; I need to make this happen,* I thought. Here, among the multitude of things I couldn't do, was something I could do with the potential for tremendous benefit.

In the weeks after meeting Haven, I strategized about raising the money to purchase her. My research revealed that $16,500 was a reasonable price for a fully trained and documented service dog, but I didn't have that kind of cash. A friend mentioned GoFundMe, and I sketched out a campaign plan; my brother, T.J., volunteered to make a fundraising video, asking me to send videos and photos of Holden and Haven. He also edited my narrative script:

"I am raising money for a service dog for my son, Holden, a seven-year-old boy in Brookings, South Dakota," I began. After describing LKS and how Holden experienced it, I talked about the service Haven could provide. "Haven will be another set of eyes on Holden when I am making dinner, a secure friend when Holden is having trouble sleeping, an icebreaker when meeting new friends, someone (besides me) to snuggle with when sad or frustrated, and a good listener to books. Plus, as a certified service dog, Haven can accompany us to our many blood draws, hospital stays, and outings."

T.J. advised me on producing good audio and made artful suggestions and edits, layering narrative and image perfectly. His video moved me to tears. But asking my brother for help was easier than asking my community; I'd never asked for money before, which carried the twin tinges of desperation and shame. *This is the material of your life now,* I told myself. *Shift into this reality and swallow your pride.*

Looking back, I understand this difficult emotional territory. In my working-class family, a person didn't ask for help except under extreme circumstances, and sometimes not even then. I'd been taught to dig in my heels and work harder or go without. Asking for help was tough because it also meant being open about Holden's disability and vulnerable to judgment from others about our circumstances. As I sent out the emails to launch the campaign, my heart pounded. I felt sick to my stomach. *Focus on Holden; it's for him,* I reasoned. Hope replaced fear when a few friends and acquaintances shared my social media posts and donated, but my anxiety about the whole endeavour remained for weeks.

In the end, the campaign yielded an outpouring of financial and emotional support, as well as increased awareness about epilepsy and LKS. And I raised more money than we needed. A friend sent me a cheque with a note: "I didn't know how to help you until I saw this. Now, at least I know I've given a little bit to show you my love and support. Thanks for this opportunity." That felt good.

* * *

Kafer's *crip time* reveals how disability affects one's orientation to time and can also refer to the phenomenon of disabled people being late for events (or starting events late). It can reflect the understanding that disabled people often need more time, or a different quality of time, to complete tasks. In other words, crip time signals flexibility. As Kafer writes, "Rather than bend disabled bodies and minds to meet the clock, crip time bends the clock to meet disabled bodies and minds."[7] Had I had this language, I could have better understood how to advocate for Holden at school.

Early on, I felt ashamed that I couldn't name good practices for teaching Holden. His first-grade teacher had described his typical day as one of movement: he bounced from the reading carpet to his desk to the whiteboard to the wall where he hung his backpack; sometimes he focused on a worksheet or manipulative used to teach math, and sometimes he'd bolt out of the room. After his diagnosis, his team amended his IEP to include a one-on-one assistant who followed Holden's lead. Sometimes they read books while the other children continued with lessons. Sometimes they kicked a ball around in the gym. Sometimes they went to the resource room—a smaller room for kids with IEPs. Sometimes they checked out the lunchroom. Trying to force Holden to stay put often led to a meltdown, so they tried to prevent them.

No one seemed to know what day-to-day classroom activities should look like for a child whose use of language fluctuated. Once, when I asked for a phone consult with Dr. Pratt, she recommended that Holden's teachers try the usual activities, but she cautioned that they shouldn't expect him to make progress. "The goal is to keep school a place Holden wants to be," Dr. Pratt said. "And to optimize his chances of success." How could one measure success for Holden? Those goals seemed so contradictory that I could hardly reconcile them.

After the summer of reorientation and shifting to crip time (without knowing I was doing so), I had a sense of how I might proceed. I met often with his new Deaf educator, Ms. Addison, who had experience teaching Deaf students but not students who needed as much support as Holden. I explained Dr. Pratt's advice to Ms. Addison and urged her to capitalize on Holden's strengths—namely activities that used muscle memory and procedural or rote learning. Her lesson plans paired ASL and verbal speech with things he knew how to do in order to build avenues for communication, which was excellent.

In one of these meetings, as I tried to find the language to explain what I hoped for Holden's school days, I landed on a concept that would interrupt progress—the educational version of the curative imaginary. I asked his teacher to replace progress with exposure. Exposure meant offering Holden learning opportunities and activities where he could engage with language, culture, people, and texts. Whatever got traction—whatever kept his attention for more than a few minutes—meant exposure. Would he remember? Maybe. Would he be able to tell us about it? Doubtful. But progress measured in the traditional ways simply set everyone up for failure.

I knew that exposure versus progress required a revision of the predominant way teachers think about their craft. Adapting the framework to think about Holden's learning was an ongoing process for me. When Dr. Pratt had said, "When LKS is active—when seizure activity is pervasive—Holden's on a learning hiatus," my mind caught on *hiatus*. Pause. Interruption. Suspension. It felt both absurd and apt. Absurd because we were talking about school—can teachers and schools even work from the premise that a child can't learn? And apt because yes, we couldn't force learning or remembering. Dr. Pratt continued, "Even if he does learn concepts, he can't always produce them for you when you ask, and probably not the way you asked." Then she landed on an analogy I'd used as well: "Sometimes Holden's brain is in a fog—a fog caused by seizures that you can only see on the EEG. When this happens, experiences may seem foggy to him later on." It wasn't about whether he wanted to learn, but if he could learn in that moment. Understanding this altered what I knew to be true about teaching: exposure to ideas and experiences might not equal stair-step mastery, but learning could still happen out of sync.

* * *

Perhaps I wasn't consciously altering my relationship with time via queer, crip-time routes, but that fall, the decisions I made felt both subversive and out of sync with the socially approved ways I'd engaged time and decision-making before.

In October, after Dr. Jones's nurse told me that Holden was not a candidate for brain surgery because the seizures originated on both sides of his brain,[8] after Dr. Jones tweaked Holden's medication cocktail (again) by adding Klonopin to address insomnia, and after I took a week to adjust our lives accordingly, Brian asked me to sync our electronic calendars. A few days later, *get married?* surfaced on mine. The day would be in the middle of a three-day weekend: Sunday, October 13. I laughed at Brian's planning. "Why not?" I replied. I wasn't in a hurry, but the weather still held a trace of warmth and Brian's apartment lease was ending later that month. The condo was being updated, and I still hadn't sold my house. We decided to run off to Minneapolis. With one week to arrange things, we got our licence in Minnesota, made hotel reservations, gathered up rings and clothes, retained an officiant, found a photographer, and asked my parents to drive up to watch Holden.

Brian and I promised to compose our lives together on a sunny afternoon in downtown Minneapolis. We selected a spot in Mill Ruins Park near the Stone Arch Bridge, a former railroad bridge that crossed the Mississippi River and the Falls of St. Anthony, the only natural waterfalls in that part of the river. Amid the remains of an industrial flour mill and a railroad's rusted girder piers, bushes pushed through cracks. Green and gold grasses grew on stone piers and brushed our shoes as we made our way to a gathering spot.

The photographer, the officiant, and our witness (the officiant's wife) met us in this urban park shortly before 4:00 p.m. I set down my bouquet, bought that morning at a grocery store, so we could hold hands. Brian's hands were strong and warm. He looked so handsome in his dark blue suit and pink bow tie, and I felt pretty in my white cocktail dress, even if a bit chilly as a cool breeze wrapped my shoulders. We both smiled a lot and cried a little as we exchanged vows—the updated traditional kind as well as ones we had written. I read "All My Engineering," the poem that held so much meaning for us, and then the officiant blessed our union.

Even though we were outside in a major city on a busy day, the world seemed quiet around us until the final moment of the ceremony, when we kissed. As the two of us lingered there, cheers and applause descended upon us. We looked up to see a crowd had gathered on the Stone Arch Bridge to watch our exchange. The private moment turned public in the best way—strangers joining us in our joy.

Chapter Thirteen

INTERFACE: a point of meeting

THAT WINTER, BRIAN, HOLDEN, AND I CELEBRATED CHRISTMAS, Holden's eighth birthday, and an offer on the house. I rolled with each change, throwing myself fully into both tasks and opportunities—the material of my life, the process of making. We squeezed the belongings of three people into the condo the third week of January, jettisoning rooms of stuff. "Keep a piece of furniture if it has quality or a story," Brian said, which made the gestalt of our merged styles eclectic. The condo's fresh paint, new bathrooms, and updated fixtures made it feel especially ours. After we arranged furniture and hung up our art, a sense of home and increased safety settled inside me. These feelings strengthened at the end of January when Haven finished her service-dog training and joined our family. When I looked around the condo, I saw what resulted from working with the now, not a far-away when.

In a lecture that Rosemarie Garland-Thomson gave at Luther College in 2022, she defines disability as "a set of stories we receive, through our acculturation, and that we remake in our lives and in our communities, about human variations that scientific medicine considers to be disability, disease, illness, and what we sometimes call bodymind differences."[1] She's wrestled away the power of scientific medicine to be the only storyteller, the only interpretive frame. She gives us the power to receive and remake, implying that stories can be affirmed, challenged, and changed. I'd also argue that they can be multiple and contradictory and fraught with the tension of ever emerging, always becoming.

By the time we'd moved into our new condo, I'd begun to story disability. I storied it to myself, my family, and my community in informal ways. In poetry and essays, I'd started to write about my relationship to disability as Holden's mom. Looking back, I see how fragmented these stories were, how raw. I see how they didn't always *remake* as Garland-Thomson suggests they can be; sometimes I circulated the narratives I'd received without much critical intervention.

The lenses I used to help me revise were the theories about storytelling that I knew well—the theories of composition. As a writer, I engage the creative act of making stories intellectually as well as practically, through recursive drafting and revision. I consciously borrowed methods from my writing process to be a better parent. Just as I did for new poems or essays, I took inspiration from experience, but in this context, I made daily logs and charts. For example, I jotted down what kinds of communication seemed to work well for Holden. I noted the parts of the day where he seemed most attentive, most relaxed. Whether he was cuddling with Haven on the couch or watching a movie, I listened for qualities of his speech. And I continued to conduct research, especially on the kinds of supports for kids with LKS, such as speech therapy. I engaged reflection and analysis to guide action.

Thinking about my parenting as a process meant I could make mistakes and try again. I could revise. It meant that I could experiment with ways to work with Holden, and if they failed, I could try another without shame because that's what I did when writing. It meant that the fluctuating quality of LKS and the way it shaped Holden's behaviour became another wrinkle in the plot of the day, a tension point I was bound to erase from my memory after reflecting upon it. I wrote my story of disability daily, and with the language of composing, revising my life felt a bit more familiar.

In my writing life, I was practising intense revision, too. I received a rejection for a poetry manuscript from a press that had invited the submission, and for a short time, I couldn't see a way through the rejection. I'd intended the manuscript to be about love. I included a love poem to Holden's two-foot-long T. rex toy, and a poem about miscarriage that featured tight-budded lilies. I compared my body to a bolster ready for lacemaking, and I compared my desire to have a child to nurturing crops. Then I crammed every single poem I'd written that could remotely be an expression of love into that manuscript. I'd assumed that a publication contract would follow. When I read the rejection letter, I wept. I complained to Brian and deflected his pep talk. I didn't want to do more work on the manuscript, and I didn't know how to tackle that kind of work if I could muster the motivation.

Several hours later, post-tantrum, I read the letter again. The series editor and the editor of the press liked individual poems, but they thought the manuscript as a whole was doing too much. *What are the stories in this manuscript?* I asked myself. As soon as Holden fell asleep that night, I printed it out and stayed up until midnight rereading it. I observed its tensions. I analyzed its themes. I considered its various strands. I sorted the "relationship" poems from the "motherhood" poems and ended up with a few odd poems that didn't fit either thematic grouping. By the end of the night, I had three-quarters of a manuscript about love and love lost and one-third of a manuscript about epilepsy, miscarriage, and mothering. Later, I would understand this as another moment of deepening my writing practice. Big, overarching revisions are another form of inquiry, another way of shifting frames, another way of producing new artwork. But just as I'd experienced in life, letting go of the original plans for a project is difficult. In both, however, revisions ushered in opportunities for growth.

As spring unfolded, I worked in my new writing spot—my office desk in the condo—to finish one manuscript. Between hiring a caregiver to help with Holden and finishing up semester grading, I arranged poems to create a narrative arc of a couple falling in love, that love unravelling, and the woman's love for herself reestablished. In June and the beginning of July, between taking care of Holden when his caregiver had summer class and tending the plants in our courtyard, I wrote a few more poems and retitled others to round out the narrative. I resubmitted the manuscript, and I received a publication contract from the University of New Mexico Press a few months later for my book *Untrussed*.

* * *

"Smile, Holden!" I snapped a photo of him giving me a thumbs-up from the back seat. In his *Star Wars* shirt and headphones, he looked as if he knew what to expect from a summer road trip. He didn't seem upset that we were leaving Haven at home under the care of a friend. We'd hoped to have full days exploring Denver, Colorado, and we didn't want to exhaust Haven or leave her cooped up in a strange hotel room either. Brian finished securing the bikes to the back of our car and we headed west. It was July, the height of heat on the Plains. Brian and I shared ideas about what we might do in Denver—swim, bike, shop—but not any expectations for when and how those activities would happen.

Just as we crossed into Nebraska, a pit stop for gas and a bathroom break revealed a challenge we hadn't anticipated. The convenience store didn't look familiar to Holden; anxiety flared. As we walked through the aisles toward the bathroom, Holden spied a bag of Skittles. We narrowly avoided a tantrum over the candy by rerouting him to the washroom.

"Next time, I'm going to let him take his iPad inside," I told Brian after getting Holden buckled in the car. "We should always have a strategy for unexpected candy sightings."

Brian nodded. "Yes. Think tactically."

Brian suggested that tactics were the actual ways to achieve an objective, as opposed to simply engaging an overall plan. Tactics emerged as flexible methods—mini procedures for manoeuvring through the bursts of extreme behaviour or seizure activity. They included ways of calming down, such as breathing deeply and focusing on the moment; lists of possible responses to Holden, both verbal and signed; patterns that we could engage; and tools to help with this work. The iPad, for example, was a tool, as was my iPhone cued up to play the Muppets' Swedish Chef popcorn shrimp video. Sometimes books could be tools. Sometimes Haven. I learned to switch tactics depending on the situation, just as I switched tools (imagery, sound, tension, lineation) when writing a poem. As with writing, tactics got easier with practice.

In Denver, biking was our go-to tactic. The three of us biked for miles and miles along Cherry Creek and Flat River paths, observing summer-creek splashers, sunbathers, and urban picnickers along the way. Holden rode on a half-bike that Brian had bought for him; it attached to the back of Brian's bike so Holden didn't need to steer, but he could pedal its one wheel. At first, I'd been nervous about the half-bike. Would Holden's erratic behaviour prove difficult to manage on the bike? What if he had a big seizure? What if he decided to jump off in the middle of the road? But after a few times riding around Brookings, we established a route—mostly bike trails with a few streets in the mix—and Holden seemed to like it once we got going. Often, he'd whine and protest even as he put on his helmet and jumped onto the bike. Sometimes he complained the whole ride, only to thank Brian afterward for "a lot of fun."

Revision happened incrementally in the way Brian, Holden, and I related to each other as an unfolding family, and, as the Denver trip illuminated, each day brought highs and lows and sometimes new tactics for moving forward. In many ways, our new life together revolved around anticipating Holden's needs and care, especially after Abel moved to Sioux Falls. Abel had said that Brookings felt increasingly small, and he wanted a fresh place. He reduced his visitation schedule from seeing Holden every other day (after school till the evening) and half of each weekend to two weekends per month. After that happened, Brian's role in Holden's life shifted remarkably. Brian became an excellent observer of Holden's seizure-related behaviour, and he helped me recognize patterns.

As we rode through Denver's downtown and farther afield in one of its park complexes, Brian told stories of living in Denver years ago. Holden hummed and recited movies. At lunchtime or snack time, we'd find a grocery store to purchase a picnic or buy takeout to eat at an outdoor table. Despite the relief these moments provided, Brian and I were never at ease. Biking wasn't always stress-free. In Brookings a few months prior, when the two of them went on a ride without me, Brian chose a route through an empty parking lot instead of down the street as we normally did. Holden protested. Brian stopped. He didn't have much practice managing Holden's meltdowns. Holden jumped off the half-bike, sat in the middle of the parking lot, and began to sob. The more Brian tried to get Holden back on the bike (home was only one block away), the more Holden resisted. As he thrashed around and yelled, Brian felt acutely on display. Then a couple in a car drove by slowly, asking Holden if he needed help. When Brian told them to mind their own business, they took photos of the two of them.

Unlike my mother, who refused to take Holden anywhere in public by herself after a similar event happened to her in Walmart, Brian kept trying to keep Holden active in the world for the same reasons I did. "Holden can't stay locked up in the house," he'd say. "We've got to try."

Other Holden-friendly activities in Denver were met with mixed results. At the aquarium, Holden roved the maze of fish tanks. Impish and impulsive, he rarely looked at sharks, corals, and starfish; he ran through exhibits willy-nilly. Women dressed as mermaids caught his attention, though, as if the shock of seeing make-believe characters was enough to penetrate the fog in his brain. At the downtown library, I encouraged him to select some books, but he just shrugged and ran down a hallway. Insomnia kept him awake two nights in a row, so much that on the second-to-last day of our trip, he fell asleep on the bike and nearly fell off. We stopped at a park and let him nap on a bench for an hour, his head on my legs and his feet in Brian's lap.

When the three of us were together, Brian most often made space for me to redirect Holden and mitigate his meltdowns because the more he tried to do so, the more Holden resisted Brian's parenting. Holden couldn't understand Brian's care—he was a new person in Holden's life, and someone who competed with him for his mother's attention. This hurt Brian. When a firm voice or repetition didn't work fast enough, sometimes Brian yelled. And that hurt Holden. Nothing worked consistently. Sometimes I yelled, even though I'd had more time than Brian to work on my patience. Brian's daughter, Carrie, had been a fairly compliant child and easy to entertain. Brian didn't have any experience with these parenting challenges.

And yet, Holden seemed to care about Brian even as he grappled with his role in his life. At the hotel pool in Denver, we swam each evening. Once, as Brian and Holden dove for pennies in the shallow end, Holden laughed at Brian's antics and called him his best friend.

On the last night of our trip, Brian suggested Lakeside Amusement Park, which was a gamble. We only had to pay per ride, though, so we could leave at a moment's notice without wasting a wad of cash. Over one hundred years old, the park felt steeped in wonder. We walked around at dusk, our heels crunching spilled popcorn as the neon signage flickered on. Brian and I took turns taking Holden on roller coasters and tilt-a-whirls. On the bumper cars, Holden actually laughed as Brian steered them between cars only to get nudged from behind. On the top of the Ferris wheel, I snapped a photo of all of us smiling.

* * *

September inaugurated the beginning of my post-tenure sabbatical, and I'd hoped to spend it writing. Earning academic tenure and promotion had felt gruelling. First, I'd organized six years' worth of evidence of good teaching (reviews, samples of student work, awards my students won), evidence of good scholarship (book publications and peer-reviewed presentations), and evidence of good service (community outreach plus serving on myriad department and university communities) into a binder. Then I analyzed it all to argue that I deserved tenure and promotion and submitted it to an outside committee of peers as well as an internal committee of SDSU colleagues. And I compiled this while newly divorced and raising Holden. When SDSU bestowed associate professor status on me, I applied for a semester off from teaching and service so I could jump-start a new writing project.

Pregnancy wasn't what I had in mind.

Holden was with his dad in Sioux Falls for the weekend. Brian was at a conference in Baltimore. I wanted to invite a friend or two over for a happy hour in my courtyard, but something stopped me from placing the calls. A nagging suspicion. My period was a few days late. And my period was rarely a few days late.

Before Brian and I got married, we'd discussed trying to have a child. Sitting in front of the Brookings Arts Council, we'd gazed at the county courthouse and his apartment building—the children's museum just over our shoulders. Arms around each other, we'd talked for a long time. By the end of that conversation, we both closed that door.

But we never closed the door in practice; our new love made us feel like teenagers, lazy and confident in our incomplete wisdom. I told myself I was now too old to get pregnant. Most women in their forties seemed to be. The chances of spontaneous pregnancy at age forty? Five percent. And I was forty-one.[2] It was probably an August afternoon, celebrating the start of my sabbatical, that we conceived.

I tore apart the bathroom searching for a pregnancy test left over from the attempts four years earlier. After the stick turned positive, I cussed and cried. I blurted the news to Brian on the phone. He was stunned. "Carrie just started university this week," he said. "You're sure, right?"

Despite his shock, Brian was ready to think about the pregnancy coming to term without question. I caught him researching genealogy sites for names associated with the Rex family, and he admitted he'd told a good friend the news. When he talked about the baby as a sure thing, I deflected. I was waiting for another miscarriage. Women between forty and forty-four have a 33 percent chance of miscarriage—and I'd already had four.[3] Those facts together made me certain the pregnancy would end early. I cancelled my participation in two international conferences for fear of miscarrying away from home. I traced the numbers in the calendar, my finger brushing each day in September and October as I wondered which day the bleeding would start. The lab workups and ultrasounds my doctor ordered to keep a good eye on the pregnancy's progression gave me jolts of excitement, but even still, I told Brian about the results in clinical terms: "My hormone levels are increasing—a good sign," I texted him. He responded positively, but I left it there.

I existed in a slump of nausea and blunted fear, vomiting one, two, sometimes three times a day. Blogs and websites said intense nausea was good, but I resisted believing. This sign had failed before. I tried to read, and I dabbled in words, but I couldn't distract myself from the body's processes of making and what I thought could be, on some days, unmaking.

And I already loved the growing potential inside of me, as I always did.

Although I tried waiting until the end of November—the beginning of the second trimester—to tell anyone, at the end of September I sobbed the news to my mother on the phone. When she advised me to pray, I responded, "I don't even know what to pray for." She answered, "Pray that you'll accept whatever happens." That advice propelled me through the days I verged on despair.

* * *

Garland-Thomson says that disability can represent "aspects of the human condition that are unpredictable, unstable, and unexpected: in short, contingency itself."[4] From my understanding of her work, she argues that if the cultural stories about disability shifted from the eugenic elimination of disability to conserving disability for its contributions to society, then more women would also be more likely to choose to continue pregnancies when genetic testing revealed the probability of disability. So often, the stories we hold shape our imaginations—our perceptions of the present reaching far into our future lives.

Unlike my pregnancy with Holden, my advanced maternal age—forty-one—existed alongside stories medical research told. Unlike my pregnancy with Holden, I was asked to make decisions. My OB/GYN offered me a test called MaterniT21, a blood test that screened for three common chromosomal differences, including trisomy 21 (Down syndrome), trisomy 18 (Edwards syndrome), and trisomy 13 (Patau syndrome). I learned that the two new to me, 18 and 13, usually ended in stillbirth or the death of the infant. I also discovered that for women who get pregnant at forty, the possibility for Down syndrome is about one in one hundred.

I'd declined testing when I was pregnant with Holden, but this time I said yes to MaterniT21. I remember rolling up my sleeve and saying, "Let's do it right now." Every stretched muscle that I interpreted as a cramp sent me to the bathroom. Every time I slid my underwear down, I expected to see blood. Anything that could curb my fear of miscarriage and help me survive the day-to-day anxiety seemed like a gift. For me, ruling out these trisomies meant ruling out miscarriage.

If I'd had the wisdom of Garland-Thomson—the framework of embracing the unexpected—it might've helped me with that first trimester. I coped rather than embraced. It wasn't the abyss that beckoned; no. This feeling was grounded in the physical: the fear tightened my chest, stifled my breathing. At night, I slept for a few hours only to be awakened by something—a dream? I never remembered, but my heart raced upon waking. Sometimes it took me hours to get back to sleep.

I never let myself think at any length about what would happen if the results indicated any of those trisomies were likely. I couldn't think, even in the tiniest way, about my baby dying, and when I thought of Down syndrome, I pictured my cousin Nancy, my great-aunt's daughter. I'd spent a good deal of time with Nancy before my grandmother passed away, and I was fond of her talent for remembering everyone's birthday and her gift for making me laugh. But really, I appreciated her willingness to talk about Theresa without any self-consciousness. Nancy knew Theresa had died, but she didn't talk about her with the same worry that she'd make me cry or cause me pain like other family members did. It felt freeing to remember Theresa with her. I recalled attending Nancy's graduation from high school in the early 1980s and my mother saying that back in her day, people with Down syndrome didn't live as long as Nancy had, and that expectations for their lives and education were far lower than what they now knew was possible. Despite these stories and experiences, I bracketed the possibility of Down syndrome with the others, ready to invest emotional energy into our imagined futures when the test results came back.

The only time Brian and I discussed what the tests screened for was when the hospital required us to consult with a panel of professionals. Brian and I met at the hospital, waiting for the nurse to call us—he on his phone reading emails, me in a fit of worry, trying to ward off nausea. When it was time, a nurse ushered us into a room and turned on the video link (the geneticists worked from the main hospital in Sioux Falls). The interview itself is dim in my memory; I remember them explaining what screening meant—nothing would be 100 percent. The question I remembered answering? *What would you do if the screening pointed to a chromosomal abnormality*? I said we didn't know, which was partly true. I couldn't fathom choosing abortion for any reason after wanting another child, after enduring the miscarriages. And yet I also knew that feelings changed when faced with facts, not hypotheticals.

I'd met only one person who knew her child wouldn't have long to live after he was born; she chose, without regret, to continue the pregnancy and spent fifteen hours with her son before he died.

"We're raising a child with a disability already," I told the panel. "We know what that means more than typical families, I think." I wasn't sure how to read the geneticists on the panel. Were they there to educate us? Persuade us? "This pregnancy was a surprise," I said. "We've not yet been married a year." Brian said something about waiting to see the results before making projections. I half expected them to make a case against abortion since this hospital had Catholic ties, but when we explained that Holden had a rare epilepsy syndrome and described its effects, the tone of the consultation shifted from neutral to serious. It seemed as if they knew we understood more than other parents they met in this context.

"That was a waste of time," Brian said afterward as we sat down in a nearby coffee shop. He sipped his latte, and I stirred my decaf chai, put off by the strong smell that I usually adored.

"It felt a bit perfunctory," I said.

Looking back, I wish I had encountered Garland-Thomson's work that would have added nuance to the term *chromosomal abnormality* bandied about by the doctors on the panel. Her work introduced me to the phrase *natural human variation.* This term challenged the binary of normal/abnormal by recognizing human difference as valuable and compatible with life. In a podcast interview with a genetic counsellor, Garland-Thomson discusses the ethics of ending a pregnancy based on the results of genetic testing. She simultaneously affirms the right of a woman to make a family that she wants and critiques the social narratives that would pressure a woman to abort a pregnancy based on the predicted disability of the child. Many disabilities tested for are consistent with natural human variation, Garland-Thomson explains. I appreciated how "natural human variation" upended narratives of defect and deformity, and how Garland-Thomson critiqued ableist narratives about the unequal value of human differences.[5]

But at the panel, we didn't have that phrase, which might've helped me articulate all this. And today, when I ask Brian if he remembers the panel, the test, or anything else about that day, he says no. I remember talking about the possibility of raising a child with the characteristics of Down syndrome at that coffee shop, though. We'd started to articulate implicit narratives. No one in Brian's family had a visible disability; he had gleaned stories from his neighbourhood, school, and church. When I think about the ways stories of disability are remade, Brian's stories were of two sorts: some in which disability didn't seem to affect the disabled person, and others in which it did. For example, one of his friends in high school, who was blind, played several musical instruments at a professional level, dated some of the most sought-after girls, and navigated school buildings using numbered footsteps. Juxtaposed with those stories were memories of the wing of his middle school where all the kids with disabilities studied and a neighbour's child with Down syndrome who didn't get the support she needed and was often seen alone and "out of control" in the yard.

I sensed Brian feared the possibility of parenting a child with Down syndrome because he only knew stereotypes and had only witnessed struggle. The stories I knew featured family members in their rich, messy, complex humanity. Even so, all of these stories seemed abstract. That's another manifestation of ableism: there aren't enough stories, not sufficient stories, not persuasive stories; this pervasive lack shapes the actual decisions parents make.

* * *

The day my results came back, I went to my OB/GYN appointment alone. After a quick listen to the strong heartbeat on the Doppler (I'd gotten past the eleven-week point by which the other fetuses had stopped growing) my doctor offered me a chair in the examining room and reported that the results revealed no chromosomal differences, at least the ones that could be tested for. I also learned I was having a boy. Feeling buoyant with happiness, I sailed out of the clinic.

On the two-minute drive home, I recalled stories I'd gathered over the years about how women broke the news to their partners about a new pregnancy or the sex of their baby. Instead of pushing them away as I had in the weeks before, I considered a few. I imagined buying a set of blue bow ties, one his size and one baby-sized. Or tying blue balloons to his bicycle parked outside the architecture building. But none of them were us, and none of them felt right. They smacked of other lives where families lived by plans, where what-happened-next was just built in, as it had been once for me. *We're tactical now,* I thought, nearly driving my car into the back of the garage. *Work with the material you have.* The results had given me hope that in May we'd welcome a baby.

I ran into the condo, expecting to find Brian at the kitchen table. He wasn't on the main floor, but his bike was in the garage, so I knew he was home. Then I heard water running upstairs. I paused at the door of the bathroom, thinking I could at least wait until he was done, but I couldn't. I pulled back the shower curtain, yelling, "We're having a boy! We're having a boy! And he's healthy!" Brian turned off the water and towelled off.

"He's healthy?" he asked as we walked over to the bed. We sat with our arms wrapped around each other. I cried happy tears into his armpit, which annoyed him a little. He hated tears.

"You get to have a boy! Now you'll have one of each," I said.

"I really don't care about that," he said. "He's healthy as far as we know. That's what matters." He pulled me closer, and I placed his hand on my belly. *Healthy* didn't mean *not disabled*; *healthy* meant less likely to die, and less likely to be born with medical conditions, such as heart defects and blood disorders, that would threaten that life. Healthy, as far as we knew. Despite acknowledging the myriad things that could go wrong, I allowed myself to feel joy.

"I can't believe we're actually going to have a baby," I said. "Our baby." He smiled weakly. He was happy, and he was worried. Not about miscarriage or about disability, though. He was worried, as I'd be soon, about how we'd handle parenting both boys together.

With this new hope, and the luck of some non-vomiting days, I went to the campus library to write. Lounging on a blue sofa, I wrote, "To My Sixth, Yet Unborn: / We've never met, but I love nonetheless / your fluttering heartbeat and fig-sized flesh." A tiny poem. A fun rhyming riff. Hope led to more hope, and with each passing day in November—and as the morning sickness subsided—I embraced the pregnancy more fully. Brian announced it to our wider circle of family and friends on social media by captioning a photo from a Thanksgiving trip: "Christine in Los Angeles, pregnant with our son."

As Garland-Thomson writes: "Disability demands that we all might imagine a subject without a future life trajectory perpetually managed in the present moment."[6] Perhaps it's a radical simplification, but I interpret that to mean *live in the present time.* Constantly trying to control a future by fixing, focusing on, or manipulating the present means missing out on what is—perhaps not even really perceiving what is. By the end of November, I felt open to the present moment, which meant my worry about my pregnancy not making it to term faded.

* * *

Telling Holden wouldn't be as subtle or simple, I thought. I fretted about how he'd react. I put it off until my bulging belly couldn't be ignored, and then I waited for a time when Holden seemed happy—for a time when the fog lifted and his thoughts seemed to be connecting.

One December evening, I pulled out the Christmas decorations from the storage space. Holden's eyes lit up when he saw them. He was in his usual spot, half sitting, half lying on the couch. Haven had her chin on the top of his head as if she were watching him play his video game on the iPad. On good days, he'd say to Haven: "Come here!" or "There's Haven," or "She's my girl. Such a good girl." Haven slept with Holden in his bed, and she snuggled with him on the couch. He filled her dog dish with food each morning and evening, rarely protesting this chore as he did nearly everything else.

Holden uncurled from Haven, put his iPad down, and walked over to a bin.

"Some of those are Brian's decorations from when he was a little boy, so be careful," I said. "They're fragile." He peeked inside, then moved to a different box and opened it.

"Lights!" He tugged tree lights out of the box.

"Do you want some for your bedroom?" I asked. He looked at me, so I took his hand and started to lead him to his room. He pulled back.

"No!" he screamed. I sighed. I knew he'd love them once they were there.

"I'll put them up for you later, then," I said. He opened a box of glass bulbs and started to hang all of them on the same three branches.

"Brian! You'd better help before Holden puts all the decorations on by himself," I said.

Brian walked into the room from the office with his laptop open. "Oh. Time for decorating?" he asked. I nodded, handing him a string of lights.

"Put some ornaments on other branches," Brian said. He moved to touch one, and Holden scowled at him, so he waited until Holden turned around before moving one to another part of the tree. As long as he didn't see Brian rearranging the ornaments, Holden didn't seem to care.

"It's almost Christmas," Holden said.

"Yes, you're right! Good job." I sniffed away the emotion that bit of speech summoned; last year he hadn't seemed to understand Christmas at all. We opened a box of ornaments my mother had crafted over the years: a cross-stitched Christmas stocking, plastic-canvas reindeer, a wooden birdhouse. There was even a ceramic candy cane that I'd painted with watercolours. We found a spot for all of them, and Brian put a pinwheel from his childhood on the tree as well. When we finished, the lights sparkled and reflected in the window, making the tree seem bigger.

"We just need some snow now," I said as the three of us stood before the tree.

Brian nodded, then left to finish whatever he had been working on before. Holden and I plopped down on the couch. My pregnant belly popped out. I could still wear some large-sized clothes, a few skirts that stretched, and sack dresses. I preferred maternity clothes because they were roomier in all the right places.

"Hey, Holden," I said. He looked at me. I pointed to my belly. "Does my tummy look bigger?" No response. I took his hand and put it on my belly. He couldn't feel the baby moving yet, even though I could sometimes, but I wanted to make it tangible. "I'm getting bigger because there's a baby in there," I said. "Baby. Baby in there."

He moved his hand back to the iPad screen. "Baby?" he asked.

"Yes. You're going to have a baby brother." He turned his head to look at my belly, then looked me in the eyes. *Good, I think he heard me,* I thought. *But did he understand?*

I remembered my dreams of giving Holden a sibling—Holden playing with a baby, making the baby laugh, tucking a blanket around its sleeper. I wasn't sure any of that was possible now. I was afraid because Brian and I didn't really know how we'd parent a newborn alongside Holden; I was afraid because I didn't know how to manage taking care of Holden and a new baby; I was afraid Holden would reject his brother or be jealous of him. Fear left me with a host of questions: Could they be left alone together in the same room? What would happen if they both needed me at the same time? Would I be able to keep them both safe? I imagined the baby crying and Holden trying to help by picking him up but dropping him; I imagined the baby crying and Holden trying to put something in his mouth and the baby choking; I imagined Holden throwing things and the baby getting hit.[7]

I wish I'd had Garland-Thomson's exhortation to imagine a "subject without a future life trajectory perpetually managed in the present," because even with our tactical reorientation, anxiety reared its head. Perhaps, if I could have viewed the anxiety simply as managing the stress and strain of change, I would have coped better. Instead, that anxiety was also still paired with the fear that I'd lose a child. In "The Case for Conserving Disability," when Garland-Thomson makes her argument about being open to the unexpected, she draws on Chris Gabbard's memoir *A Life Beyond Reason* as well as Emily Rapp's *The Still Point of a Turning World*. In both, the writers' disabled children die. Garland-Thomson offers a reading of these two books as a gift of knowledge and cultural production that shows disability as an ethical resource: "[P]eople with disabilities and disability in general present the difficult challenge ... to engage in a relationship not based on the promise of the future."[8]

I couldn't help but think of my own mother, who had endured the death of my sister, Theresa. I knew she wouldn't trade those twenty years of life to erase the pain of death. I knew she still missed Theresa, even as she laughed over some funny comment my brother made, even as she hugged Holden and held him close.

Sitting there next to Holden on the couch, my new logic countered tactical thought. Perhaps not the radical remaking that Garland-Thomson argued for, but my approximation: how well the boys would get along, and how well I'd be able to keep them safe, was unknown. Time would pass and the baby would come, and then I'd be closer to knowing how this unexpected gift would change us all.

Chapter Fourteen

INTERDEPENDENT: mutually dependent

IN "UNDERSTANDING DISABLED FAMILIES: REPLACING TALES of Burden and Resilience with Ties of Interdependency," Janice McLaughlin refers to families with disabled members as *disabled families* because "the family as a whole ... live and experience disability."[1] Indeed, communities respond to families differently due to disability. I had conceptualized this long before I read about it. Reflecting on the ways Holden's disability had influenced my routines, my engagement with public spaces, and how my professorial work happened, I had thought: As Holden's mom, does this mean that society disables me? Do its narratives create barriers for me because of our relationship? But I hadn't encountered anyone who actually made that argument until I found McLaughlin's chapter in a disability textbook. McLaughlin interprets the ways families report their battles with social institutions for services: the problems aren't with the disabled child but with accessing support for that child. Resisting the dominant narrative of burden, McLaughlin replaces it with interdependency, recognizing that our lives are intertwined to various degrees with others. In a disabled family, all members are full and valued participants in family life.[2]

In May, Brian, Holden, and I welcomed a new member to our family, and I began to see a new degree of interdependency—a new manifestation of how intertwined we had become.

* * *

On the third of May, my forty-second birthday, I puttered around the space Brian and I had made in our bedroom for the baby. I put sheets with green polka dots on the crib, a green-striped cover on the changing table, and a cover on the rocking-chair pillow. On the wall of shelves, I opened drawers and refolded onesies and sleepers. On the fourth of May, after conducting two classes and eating dinner, I stayed up late restacking diapers, double-checking the security of the mobile, and recounting the number of receiving blankets. Brian and Mom had suggested I go to bed early since the C-section was scheduled for 7:00 a.m. the next morning, but sleep eluded me. I lay there, feeling my baby move around. I tracked his hiccups, which he usually got twice a day, before finally succumbing to sleep.

Then I dreamed of Theresa. The two of us were going out to brunch with her friend; we slid on lipstick, primping in front of the mirror together. The prospect of talking to her after all those years thrilled me, but just as we turned to leave, she stopped. A door opened and her friend walked through it. "You can't go out to brunch with us, Christine," she said. "You need to take care of the baby." I turned to find Theresa holding a swaddled infant, and she put the baby in my arms without a word. When she looked into my eyes, her beauty—blue eyes, glowing skin, megawatt smile—stunned me. I woke up, happy and heartbroken, feeling pressure on my arms.

Xavier Stewart Rex was born at 7:45 a.m. on May 5. Brian snapped photos of Xavier getting weighed before bringing him over to me. Xavier had stopped crying, apparently mesmerized by the lights in the room, and once Brian put him against my chest, he squeaked and squirmed, already ready to eat. Xavier had a mess of brown hair, which surprised me, since both Brian and I were born bald or wispy blond. His face was round like mine. In my favourite photo of that morning, Brian's holding Xavier, his new-dad expression a mix of pride and shock.

That afternoon, I photographed my two sons. When my mom brought Holden to the hospital, he looked at the IV and walked right over to me, an expression of concern on his face.

"I'm okay," I said. "Here's your brother."

Holden stepped next to Xavier, swaddled on my bed. Brian got up from his chair and stood at the foot of the bed, alert and waiting. "This is Xavier," I continued.

Holden's eyes widened and he smiled. "Here, give him your finger. He'll grab it." Holden's energy was calm, gentle. He didn't resist when I unfolded one of his fingers and slid it into Xavier's hand; Xavier grasped it. I opened my phone camera in my other hand.

"Isn't he so sweet and tiny?"

Holden nodded, bending down to kiss him on the forehead; his lips touched Xavier's hair. I snapped a photo, which broke the moment. Holden scooted down on the bed and looked back at his iPad. I looked up at Brian, and he smiled at me.

* * *

Looks-wise, no one could tell these two were brothers—half brothers, but I never use that term. After a few months, blond wisps replaced Xavier's brown hair. His eyes were the same blue as mine but the exact intensity and shape as Theresa's—more widely set and more luminous. As he grew, we'd see that his expressions were Brian's: grin, smirk, "I'm concentrating" look. Xavier's nose was mine: a regular sort, not too wide, not too thin, rather round. Holden, with his dark brown hair, deep-set brown eyes, and full lips, was Xavier's opposite.

Affection-wise, everyone could tell these two were brothers. When he was feeling good, Holden doted on Xavier. And if Holden was in the room, Xavier had him in sight. Holden often asked to hold Xavier, but after a few minutes, he'd announce, "This baby is too squirmy!" That suited curious Xavier, who was always ready to move and play.

Xavier's presence required revised routines. Even getting the basics in—fresh air, a bit of exercise, grocery shopping, meal prep—shifted.

I couldn't take Xavier and Holden outside because if Holden ran ahead, I couldn't move fast enough with the baby to follow him. If Holden had a meltdown, I couldn't tend to both boys. That summer, I hired a caregiver to provide a second set of hands and eyes when Brian was working, but during the first week I took her to the grocery store with us and Holden had a tantrum, throwing a loaf of bread and a can of tomatoes out of the cart. She quit that night. We spent a lot more time in the condo watching screens than I'd hoped to that summer. Between nursing and changing Xavier and feeding and tending to Holden, activities I wanted to pursue—like exercise and writing—fell off the list.

Slowly, Brian and I learned that Holden could participate more fully in family life if we gave him big-brother responsibilities. One morning, the four of us ventured out to a café for breakfast. I'd packed Holden's iPad and a few books for Xavier, which Holden spied in the bag as we sat down. He wanted the book *Good Night, Gorilla*. He'd owned that one years ago.

"Read it to your brother," I said to Holden, scooching Xavier's car seat around so the two were next to each other. Holden set the book on top of the menu and opened it. He named all the animals and said good night on each page. A few times, he pointed out a few details in the pictures as I had done for him.

"Keys!" he said, smiling at Xavier. "Oh no!" he exclaimed as all the animals left the zoo. Xavier looked at the book and then looked at his brother. For a few minutes they interacted like this—a tiny slice of time that created a pathway for a stronger bond as they grew. As we added a few responsibilities to Holden's repertoire, we learned that they could distract him from his usual patterns and create new possibilities. If we did venture out, I asked Holden to push the stroller or cart, which he enjoyed. He also began to teach Xavier about his favourite superheroes, naming each when he saw them pass over the screen of his iPad.

* * *

I recognized from the moment Xavier and Holden met that their lives would intertwine and that each of them would be better for it. That notion, sparked by how the two responded to each other, counters the dominant narrative of disability as burden. McLaughlin explains that in the literature on siblings of disabled children, "the dominant voice and concern has revolved around non-disabled children whose lives are disrupted" by a disabled family member.[3] They are described as maturing too quickly due to caregiving responsibilities, which makes them resentful. McLaughlin resists these assertions, illuminating my experience. Once I understood that Holden would be careful around his infant sibling, I shifted my framework and saw the positive influences Holden could have on Xavier and vice versa.

By the time Xavier was a toddler, he perceived Holden as a big brother ready to play—even when he wasn't—and he pulled language from Holden like a magician pulling handkerchiefs from their sleeve:

"Mom! Xavier's crying."

"Mom! Xavier put a LEGO in his mouth."

"Mom! Xavier's attacking me with his baby hand."

"Mom! Xavier has a stinky D."

He put his communication efforts into helping, into keeping Xavier safe. And Xavier kept Holden on his toes. Even when he didn't want to leave his iPad for a moment, Xavier developed persuasive tools. Once, Xavier grabbed a plastic container from the spice drawer, took it into the living room, and sprinkled his brother with it.

"Mom! Xavier's got paprika!"

I burst out laughing. Sure enough, Xavier and Holden were covered in red spice. I didn't know what amazed me the most: that Xavier had stretched far enough to grab the container, or that Holden knew that it was paprika. Had he read the label? We'd never talked about paprika before.

The first time Xavier elicited non-screen play from Holden surprised me. Xavier was about ten months old, and I'd found some of Holden's Hot Wheels cars and tracks that he hadn't played with in years. When Holden saw me trying to show Xavier how to push the cars down the tracks, he joined in by making one long track that went down the hallway from one end of the condo to the other. Holden explained to Xavier: "Connect the tracks." They crashed two cars in the middle, and they laughed and laughed. When Xavier tried to take the tracks apart, Holden stopped him.

"No, no, brother."

Holden insisted on crashing the cars over and over, resisting any other way to play.

"Look! Race this way," I said.

But it didn't matter to me that Holden wouldn't change things up. My sons were playing, and they were playing together.

One afternoon I asked Holden to accompany me to pick up Xavier from daycare. He refused at first, but when I gave him his iPad, he tossed it into his backpack and followed me into the car. Holden spent the four-minute drive reciting scenes from *Scooby-Doo* mashed with *The Muppet Movie.* I tried to engage him with questions, but he ignored them.

"Put your iPad under your arm, please," I told Holden once we arrived at the centre. He did. Once through the doors, Holden beelined to Xavier's room.

"There he is! Baby brother!"

He pointed at another blond boy first; sometimes it took him a few seconds to recognize Xavier among other children. Once Xavier saw Holden, he ran over to us, grinning. Holden opened the door and hugged Xavier. Xavier returned the squeeze.

"I found him! I found Xavier!"

Holden's voice bounced off the centre's walls.

"Inside voice, please," I said. I turned to Xavier. "Say goodbye to teachers and friends."

"Bye! Bye!" Xavier said. Holden echoed him and he grabbed Xavier's hand. Xavier wiggled out. After months of watching and listening, Holden understood the need to keep Xavier safe. My two boys walked together down the hall, Holden with his iPad under one arm, his other extended to Xavier's hand.

As we got to the centre's door, Xavier ran ahead.

"Mom! He's loose!" Holden yelled as Xavier squeezed through the open door.

I caught up and put my hand on Xavier's head. "Walk, please," I said. The three of us walked to the car, Xavier babbling away and Holden complaining that Xavier was too loud.

Xavier was a bit of a miracle for me and a bit of a miracle for Holden.[4]

* * *

If Xavier's birth gave Holden the new role of brother, his arrival also marked a shift for me—although the agency I began to assert seems more like an ongoing response to reorientation than the direct result of Xavier's entrance into our lives. McLaughlin notes that disabled families redefine themselves across time, and those who see their disabled child as bringing value often shift their perspectives on medical interventions—an area I began to think more critically about.[5] Although I didn't refuse certain medical practices, as she found families often doing, I began to renegotiate elements. For example, I asserted my role as a parent who could provide the Minnesota Epilepsy Group with observational data; I also stepped back from expecting that their solutions would return Holden to the trajectory he'd been on before the seizures started. In these ways, I balanced advocating for Holden's safety with accepting that disability would be an enduring part of our family's reality.

By the beginning of fourth grade, Holden could sometimes express his needs in one-sentence statements, but he didn't take turns in conversation. Seizure activity still affected his receptive language ability. Because not much had changed for Holden in terms of seizure activity or language and academic skills, one of the neurologists at MEG, Dr. Olson, suggested a six-week "burst-dose" trial of steroids and the addition of a new anti-epilepsy drug, Keppra. Because specialists thought that the seizures were autoimmune in nature, steroids helped reduce them, though they didn't always end them. The burst-dose regimen often helped kids, but sometimes they regressed when the trial ended. And the higher doses of prednisone couldn't be sustained because of side effects such as an increased risk of infections, osteoporosis, and suppressed adrenal gland hormone production. I agreed with Dr. Olson regarding the trial but also clarified that I would monitor Holden's sleep, behaviour, and language closely during this period, and that my data would be part of deciding whether it worked or it didn't.

Although I'd been providing some observations before, I created a system of analysis. Every day, Holden's teacher gave me a sheet documenting his activities, including academic subjects covered and his attitude. She noted when he was sleepy, when he "refused" to participate, when he seemed depressed, etc. I analyzed the weeks before, during, and after the burst-dose trial and added my own observations from home. My goal? To see what kinds of changes the medication experiment yielded. It was clear that the Keppra increased Holden's irritability, but his ability to engage in learning increased too: he started to read a few words, his verbal expression expanded, and he learned ASL slightly faster, too. When I gave the results to the team, Dr. Pratt joked that I had pursued the wrong kind of doctoral degree; my contributions led to a more in-depth understanding. I wanted to contribute what I could to their decision-making and then accept what happened as a result. When the burst-dose regimen of prednisone ended, Holden went back to the pulse-dose regimen and experienced a few slow regressions, but never back to the pre-burst-dose level. Until the seizures that resulted in LKS disappeared during puberty, the team prescribed the burst dose twice, and both times it boosted his academic and language skills slightly.

My confidence also helped me grapple with the different kinds of medical interventions introduced alongside the burst-dose regimen. Dr. Pratt decided that Ritalin was worth trying to mitigate Holden's impulsivity, since it often sparked dangerous activity—like opening the car door while the car was moving. Ritalin worked as prescribed, but it also curbed his appetite too much. I had to research ways to get him the most calories possible with very few bites of food. A solution for one symptom always seemed to create another issue. At one point, Holden took eight different prescriptions and over-the-counter medications: two for general seizures, one for sleep, one to fight the inflammation assumed to cause the pervasive subclinical seizures, one for attention and impulsivity, melatonin to help him get to sleep, fish oil to boost brain function, and Miralax to counter chronic constipation.

With each medication addition, deletion, or dose change, my emotions surged. Change meant a risk of breakthrough seizures, more insomnia, or more intense meltdowns and tantrums. But it could also mean a decrease in seizure activity. Early on, I'd resented this power the doctors seemed to grant me over my son's care. I wasn't a medical doctor—how could I contribute to these decisions? They seemed to think in solvable algorithms, with solutions broadly applicable. My contributions felt distilled to Holden's observable patterns alone, but after shifting my perspective, I saw the value they held, and honestly—the team seemed pleased to have them. The data I contributed were simple additions to a complex equation that helped the team pivot and shift to Holden's context. Since I had moved my role to a different part of the process, my expectations for communication with them changed. I no longer hoped to hear them reflect aloud about how they solved these complex equations. I accepted the way they worked and waited to hear their suggestions or solutions. Then I used my tactics to respond to any challenges in Holden's behaviour that ensued.

* * *

Even though we saw brighter spots in learning, Holden's behaviour still perplexed me and affected our daily lives. The spitting, kicking, and hitting episodes had ended, but rigidity remained. A lack of flexibility kept him locked in the status quo, and it took what felt like Herculean feats to break him out. In the morning, I had to give him a piggyback ride from his bed to the bathroom. If we had to run an errand, I had to put on his coat for him and allow him to bring his iPad along. The routines that helped Holden make transitions and tamp down impulsivity also created their own issues. For example, the only way I could get us through the grocery store without filling my cart with mountains of junk food (that either Holden would demand loudly or put in the cart himself) was to allow Holden to select a Lunchables pack in the last store aisle. Every. Single. Store. Visit. Sometimes he didn't even eat what I secretly called his boxed bribe. This rigidity would persist for years. And sometimes, when this sidetracked an experience I got frustrated, but over time I began to see this as part of the dynamic process of parenting Holden.

One of the ways I redefined my perspective regarding Holden's future was to look elsewhere for narratives about LKS. Like most medical professionals I'd come to know, Holden's care team seemed to prefer to work with the body and with data; they didn't want to hear about my sleepless nights and disrupted plans. When the disease contributed to such profound changes for families, they couldn't prescribe solutions to fix stress, depression, or divorce. Unlike less rare kinds of medical conditions or disabilities, in-person support groups for LKS didn't exist, but I did find a group on social media. Although the list had only six or seven posts when I first stumbled upon it, it had grown to several separate groups in just over seven years.

Once a week or so, I'd sit down at my kitchen table, take a sip of chai, and start scrolling through the conversations. In my early forays into the discussion board, I'd hoped to find stories of kids who experienced a trajectory of LKS similar to Holden's. Dr. Jones had resisted looking into his crystal ball (he claimed he didn't have one), but some story out there, I reasoned, could tell me what came next for Holden. Most often, parents of newly diagnosed children would post questions about medication, and other parents, who spoke like experts, would answer in detail. Hannah's dad, for example, could explain the differences among medication protocols, and he clarified what neurologists couldn't seem to find the words for—and he did this without judgment or giving direct advice, which I admired. When parents like Poli's mom, a behaviour troubleshooter, chimed in, I put down my tea and took notes. She often had good insight regarding what worked with her son. Other parents took on lofty ambitions: Josh's mom started a research foundation and shared ideas on how to raise awareness about LKS/CSWS/ESES. Sometimes I'd post a question or answer someone's query, but I often didn't feel like I knew enough to give details. By the time I drained my mug of tea, I'd be done reading the posts. Just like Holden, few of these children ever found a clear-cut route to recovering their pre-seizure trajectory.

Over the years, I read less to see what happened next and more with an eye to help à la disability doula. And I began to see patterns. Overwhelmed by a new diagnosis, most new families wanted to know what medication protocols worked to stop the seizures. Almost everyone wanted a clear path forward. Most parents posted what medications they tried; some even posted EEG data. I saw the wide variety of ways neurologists across the country—even the world—tackled this disease; many families, like mine, had to search for a doctor with the right expertise. But when the medication couldn't halt the seizures, the stories centred on sadness, grief, and desperation. These stories were—and continue to be—a source of pain for me. I want to challenge the ways these families frame what's happening to their child; I want to offer them my insight. But it's nearly impossible to do in a discussion-board post. It's nearly impossible to persuade parents to move from a medical framework to a disability framework when they believe the only solution lies in a medication cocktail—if they can only find which one.

Two or three times a year, a parent or adult who'd survived LKS would share a story about leading an independent life, attending university, and getting married.[6] Reading these, I'd wonder if Holden would post his own someday, and I imagined a few different versions. I no longer held either of us to a Plan. Instead, I plumbed the discussion boards for insights that might help Holden flourish: activities, IEP- and school-related ideas, etc. Even though I found it a challenge, I began to see the reality that only Holden held the answers to what his life would look like, and that he would unfold it for us as he could and when he was ready.

* * *

The summer after Holden completed fourth grade and Xavier turned one, Brian and I decided to reprise the road trip vacation through Nebraska to Colorado. On a similarly hot July day, we strapped the bikes to the back of the car again, this time with an orange seat for Xavier to ride with me. I researched a list of Colorado towns that boasted good bike trails and made them possible destination points. If one place worked more than another, we conjectured, we might stay an extra night. If it didn't, we'd bail for another town on the list. We'd revise as we went.

In Valentine, Nebraska, we rode our bikes from the hotel parking lot toward a crushed-gravel bike path dubbed the Cowboy Trail. I felt uneasy. The length of the trail was much farther than I'd ridden before with Xavier on the back. Perhaps I wasn't fit enough to make this happen, I thought. Even though Holden's tantrums had started to wane, the possibility one could erupt at any moment remained. As we passed outside of town, the scene of two men on horseback working a herd of cows surprised me and delighted both boys. Xavier kept pointing at them, and Holden stared with an amused expression on his face. As we crossed the narrow Valentine Railroad Bridge—repurposed for biking since being abandoned by trains in 1992—I seemed to be the only one terrified of the height. A quarter mile long, the 148-foot-high bridge spanned the Niobrara River. The views of Nebraska—green around the river but more arid as I looked toward the horizon—distracted me with their beauty and seemed to enchant Holden, too. When Brian snapped a photo of us under a "Welcome to Valentine, Nebraska" sign, Holden's wide smile looked sincere.

McLaughlin argues that, like disabled individuals experience stigma, disabled families do as well, and that stigma can encourage a disabled family to try to appear "normal." And yet her research also points to examples where families resist narratives of normalcy and recognize their children "outside of medical and social expectations."[7] I signed Holden up for Special Olympics (swim and bowling only—he hated track and field); I entered his photographs in art competitions (special artist category); I submitted a photographic self-portrait for publication in a disability magazine (my poem accompanying his photograph); and I signed him up for another summer of horseback riding in a program for disabled youth and adults in Brookings. As McLaughlin writes, I was finding new ways of being a family that incorporated Holden's "identity and agency"[8] into what I valued and celebrated. Finding ways to fold Xavier into activities extended those practices, and the work Brian did to include Holden on bike rides and trips was also part of finding ways to be a family.

In Colorado, we often biked in the morning and took a "nap car ride" to a nearby destination in the early afternoon; Xavier surrendered to sleep best in the car. In Fort Collins, we biked around the campus at Colorado State as well as the downtown area before packing up our stuff and heading two hours to take a train ride in the mountains. In Steamboat Springs, we took the boys to a pool fed by natural hot springs, biked along the Yampa River with dozens of kayakers to entertain us along the way, and managed to stick our heads into a few shops along Lincoln Avenue without meltdowns ensuing. The day before we returned to South Dakota, Brian and I decided to try a hike. We rolled into the overflowing parking lot at Fish Creek Falls mid-morning.

"Do we have to get out here?" Holden whined as I unbuckled Xavier from his car seat.

"We're going hiking," I said. Holden complained while we gathered sunblock and a few water bottles from our stash of provisions. He'd never been on a hike in mountains before. The paved trail wound into dense pine forest, which seemed to intrigue Xavier, and he seemed unfazed by the crowd.

"Let's see this waterfall," Brian said, taking Xavier by the hand. Brian's enthusiasm for this idea surprised me. Despite his love of biking, he liked being outdoors in urban areas best. Raw nature unnerved him a bit, I imagined, with few places for his analytical-architectural mind to land. And hiking wasn't an activity someone with an artificial, often arthritic knee tended to embrace.

When that hike only took twenty minutes of easy walking, we decided to try another trail through a forest to the upper falls. I grabbed the baby backpack from my bag and clipped it on. Brian picked up Xavier and slipped him in.

"We can always turn around if it gets too tough," Brian said as we joined the other dozen hikers beginning the ascent.

Brian led our group along the dirt path, which started wide but quickly narrowed, hiking at a pace his knee allowed. I watched Holden's sneakers crunch pine needles on the forest floor, chunks of lichen-covered canyon under our feet. I assumed I had only a few minutes of hiking before Holden refused to continue, so I took in the details: how the pine and aspen shielded his face from the hot sun, the flex in his leg when his body pivoted around boulders in the path. I pointed out a fallen tree with gnarled bark. Holden looked but didn't acknowledge me. Xavier chatted in my ear in his baby way. I kept checking his head with my hand to see if he'd chucked his hat off somewhere along the trail.

Thirty minutes in, sweat dripped down my back and accumulated around the band of the backpack. Brian turned around.

"Can you believe this?" he asked, pointing to Holden. I shook my head no. Holden hiked past Brian, charging ahead up the mountain. I'd never witnessed Holden respond to anything like that before. Focused. No whining. No complaining. He enjoyed being in the moment.

We followed the switchbacks up and up and emptied our water bottles in the first forty-five minutes. Folks coming back down the mountain assured us that the upper falls and Long Lake weren't too much farther. Later I would learn that the upper falls were about 2.5 miles and 1,600 vertical feet of strenuous climbing, with a few miles of gradual meadows along the way. My legs hadn't yet started to burn, but I could feel my back complaining; Xavier added an extra twenty pounds.

Despite being out of shape for such a hike, my body seemed to remember its history of hiking—Camelback Mountain when I lived in Arizona, the Taurus Mountains when I lived in Türkiye. As the mountain drew Holden up, and Brian, Xavier, and I scrambled behind, I considered what his body remembered: soiled blankets, seizures in ditches, needles, Velcro boards; spiral shells near the sea, apple-picking, baby snuggles, baking cookies. Holden didn't know the hours of research I'd conducted, the myriad tactics I'd developed to keep him safe, nor the number of arguments I'd devised on his behalf, so I imbued all of that into my gaze when I looked at him, and I wrapped it into my touch when we hugged. A body remembers pain, and it remembers how it is loved.

Holden hiked and hiked and hiked that day. He hiked past Brian's aching knee. He hiked past empty water bottles—the ones we brought and those given to us by empathetic hikers on their way down. He hiked for nearly two hours until we came to a point where we could take off our shoes and wade in a cold stream. I changed Xavier's wet diaper and he and Brian splashed around in the creek. We told Holden this was the end—although we likely had another thirty minutes of hiking to reach the pinnacle—and that we needed to go back down.

The heat of the afternoon brought out flies, and he complained about them the whole way down the mountain, but Brian and I couldn't get over Holden's determination to hike and how the forest had absorbed his attention. And we couldn't get over how his body simply did the hike without training or cardio prep to accomplish it. I'd overthought Holden's challenges, knowing all the ways they could erupt and stall, but since the LKS had taken hold, I hadn't yet felt amazed by something Holden could do. Possibility inserted itself in my thoughts once more. What else could he do? What else would he do?

The story of that day was spotting wildflowers and waterfalls. It was Xavier on my back and Holden hiking with his Mario Kart backpack (iPad inside) up the mountain. It was Brian, in his turquoise T-shirt, managing the pain in his knee as he walked a few steps behind. That trip, that day, that hike—we revised as we went. And Holden astonished us.

* * *

I took Holden by the hand and tugged him up the ramp of the South Dakota Art Museum just a few weeks after we got back from Colorado. Sunny and warm, the weather reminded me of his first day of kindergarten five years before in the building just across Sylvan Green.

I brought Holden to the art museum because I wanted to show him something special—"something that has to do with you," I told him. I led him toward the northmost gallery featuring my exhibit, *Woman Working from Women: A Poetry Ekphrasis*. The exhibit was the visual component of three achievements: *Untrussed* and *Bluewords Greening*—my twin books—were published, too. They'd been conceived together, nurtured separately, and then published by different presses and within days of each other. The exhibit contained poems from both collections.

"Holden, look at the beautiful paintings. And my poems are next to them—poems I wrote." I extended my arm, and my hand touched a poem on the wall. Holden took a step back with our hands held, my body becoming a bridge between the art and its subject. "See your name?" I pointed to it in the poem. He relaxed and took two steps forward.

"H-O-L-D-E-N," he said. "Holden!" He smiled.

"Yes, that poem is about you!" I said. "It's called 'Art of the Body,' and I describe you being in the art museum with me. You were just a little boy, running from room to room." He looked at me blankly, as if I'd lost him trying to evoke that memory. "Can I get a picture of you next to your poem?" He nodded. I moved him closer to the piece and my poem. He smiled, head tilted down and shoulders hunched.

I didn't expect Holden to be impressed with my work or the art. When visiting museums before, I prompted him to take photos of what he saw, hoping that exposure to art and opportunities to take photographs would help him reveal the way he experienced the visual world. I never knew for sure what Holden saw, but his creative engagement with the world on his good days showed me his ability underneath the fog of

LKS. I wanted to help him stay connected to that. I wanted him to sense my love for him. I wanted to share my pride with him, too. Most of all, perhaps against odds, I hoped he'd remember his name on a museum wall and understand that he was art-worthy, special in a different sense of the word than was usually applied to him.

On the walls of the rectangular gallery, I could see reflections of the past six years brought together. "After It's Over" conjured the divorce: "When his eyes hint / anger, I blink and feel no pleasure." "Unintended Consequences" spoke to the aftermath: "In time, new shoots / will sprout even if you pray / otherwise." In "Conjuring Practice" I read my doubts about whether I would conceive again: "will I find a planted canvas in the drifts?" and in "Gladiolus," I read the miscarriages. I recalled Holden's LKS diagnosis in "Boy at Rest" as well as my new relationship with language and art in "Visual Thinking Strategies": "This means nothing rhymes / with orange, means a lexicon / of springs / means Still Life / with Limes and Grapefruit." Even my relationship with Brian was represented in "Beginning": "Here's a new grid, / a fresh space: the crisscrossed lines / that mark my lover's skin." With these windows into some of the deepest parts of my life on these walls, I felt more exposed than usual. These paintings and poems revealed my processes of revision. I stood there, reminded by my choices and words from "Lithography": "Son, you resist / my moves, my words, but in my view / we're art *because* of what life puts us through."

It felt strange to see so many fragments of my life represented in this space, but I also sensed how I'd changed. In the span of a decade, I went from being the mother of a typically developing child to the mother of a child with chronic illness to the mother of a child with a disability. My perspective shifted in subtle and profound ways. For example, I knew Holden's resistance to a new activity often emerged from anxiety sparked by transitions; once he moved through that, he usually enjoyed whatever experience I'd managed to coordinate. This understanding helped me cultivate an appreciation for inclusion. In my teaching, in my relationships, in my work, I felt more ready to give up the illusion of control, or at least confront the illusion outright. I appreciated experiences for the processes they unfurled, not the products gleaned at the end. A continuous reorientation replaced The Plan; discernment replaced just-what-happens-next. I had more tactics for the ever-unfolding present. This change of values felt profound.

As we walked around the exhibit, it felt like a ring in the spiral had come around, and a new ring had begun: patterns always mean and patterns can always break; four recurrent miscarriages didn't mean a fifth; a cogent sentence emerged after a string of echolalia; a bike ride displaced hours of watching screens. In the new ring, my relationship with my family—Holden, Brian, and Xavier—didn't feel easier. Nothing was fixed. Xavier's presence didn't eclipse the ache of the miscarriage, although it did distract from it. My marriage compelled time, attention, and ample space for revision. Holden was still having seizures, and parenting him still felt intense. And yet. Everything felt a bit lighter from an emotional point of view. Change wasn't coming as fast, and I had better methods for the process of change.

"Let's go!" Holden said, pulling me off the seat where I'd been taking in the exhibit. I smiled, and Holden led us out into the bright sunshine.

Epilogue

INTERLUCENT: shining in the midst of other things

MY READING OF "WELCOME TO HOLLAND," A FAMOUS PIECE penned in 1974 by disability rights advocate Emily Perl Kingsley,[1] is a good analog for my relationship to disability. What began with a superficial understanding shifted into confusion and ended with respect and appreciation. Kingsley's piece compares the experience of learning the unexpected news that one's child has a disability to receiving the unexpected news that one's plane will land in Holland after a much-anticipated trip to Italy. The first time I encountered "Welcome to Holland," Holden was still a typically developing toddler. When one of my students used the piece to frame her relationship to disability (she was the daughter of a mother with multiple sclerosis and a sister of a woman with cerebral palsy), she reported that her mother took profound comfort in Kingsley's words, and so did she. I annotated my student's essay with stars: "If you spend your life mourning the fact that you didn't get to Italy, you may never be free to enjoy the very special, the very lovely things ... about Holland." With my passport stamped with entries and exits from Japan, Türkiye, India, France, Greece, and

Germany, the traveller metaphor worked for me. I'd often brag that my definition of adventure meant travelling to a country where I didn't speak the language. After reading my student's essay and Kingsley's piece, I remember thinking, *The key to raising a kid with special needs is a simple shift of perspective, an adjustment to a temporary detour.*

By the time Holden was seven and had developed LKS, my relationship to disability had changed. I whispered, "Fuck Holland!" whenever someone reshared Kingsley's piece in a group I followed on social media. It wasn't Holland—Holden's diagnosis or his disability—that frustrated me, that exhausted me. It wasn't grieving my trip to Italy that overwhelmed me. Due to LKS's diverse and changing manifestations, this neurological disorder lacked a map, and I was angry that other parents got a flight plan at least. Instability was its stable condition. I arrived in Singapore at noon, only to watch it morph into Papua New Guinea at dinnertime. When I prepped for Dhaka, I wound up in Toronto. A morning that started in Paris ended in Baghdad. I had to keep my kid alive, thriving, and educated in each city. At least the climate was decent in Holland. At least one could learn Dutch over time.

Even though I'd begun to frame Holden's seizure disorder as a disability, too much change and intense parenting made it hard for me to fully appreciate what that meant. It wasn't until the medical system released us—when Holden was declared "free" of the pervasive seizures in the fall of 2019—that I saw a glimmer of wisdom in "Welcome to Holland."

After one night of data collection in St. Paul Children's Hospital, Dr. Jones walked into Holden's room with a smile.

"As you probably could tell due to the ways his verbal and academic skills have progressed, his EEG looks much better," Dr. Jones said. I felt a surge of happiness and a wave of tears; seven years was a long time to wait to hear those words. A snapshot of the EEG showed repeated patterns of brain waves that seemed regular and even, especially when juxtaposed with the EEG images saturated with seizure activity. Dr. Jones was right; we'd assumed changes were happening because sentences and even bits of conversation popped up here and there. To have it confirmed with data, though, felt supremely satisfying.

"So what happens now?" I asked, poised to take notes.

"We'll wean the prednisone and clonazepam, but keep him on the ethosuximide and lamotrigine for now. I'll get the nurse to write out that schedule for you," he said. I nodded. Dr. Jones nodded back. I expected him to say more regarding what changes Holden would now undergo. The seizures might be ending, but that didn't mean other cognitive processing issues had ended—at least not that I could tell. A pamphlet on the major sites in Holland would have been appreciated.

"Holden won't have to come back in for an EEG unless you see regression," he said. "He'll just come in for clinic visits." It felt like Dr. Jones was breaking up with us. Even if Holden's learning could now take hold without seizures wiping away new ideas every night, what kinds of support might he need? And how would I argue for that support without Dr. Pratt's neuropsychological tests and reports? And what about his "behaviour"? Holden needed help grappling with rigidity, which I was starting to understand as akin to anxiety, but I didn't understand how I could guide him through processing his big emotions.

"Who will help Holden recover his learning?" I asked.

"That will be the school's responsibility," Dr. Jones said. He meant that it had been his job to try to stop the seizures, and his job was done. I wondered if I could muster the confidence in the Brookings School District's ability to earnestly tackle Holden's unique blend of strengths and struggles.

Both grateful and confused, I stumbled to thank Dr. Jones. The right words refused to flow gracefully from my mouth. But as he closed the door with a soft thud, I felt a clarity in my new relationship to disability. I moved from being the mother of a child with a chronic health condition and disability to being the mother of a child with an intellectual disability. My heart pounded a bit harder in my chest. This understanding felt as profound as cracking ice on a frozen river or an airplane rerouted mid-flight. I finally knew what Holland looked like.

When I'd read "Welcome to Holland" the first time, I'd been wrong that a parent of a disabled child only needed a perspective shift; they needed a perspective characterized by fluency with change. For several months after that last visit with Dr. Jones, I wondered if I'd ever trust what I'd learned about living tactically. I wondered if living the process would ever feel as second nature as living according to The Plan. Italy became Holland, and although that felt profound, it didn't feel *enough*. I needed more stories, new theories, and fresh-to-me strategies.

* * *

I'd started writing *Silence and Seizure* in December 2014 when Holden was eight years old. My friends in my creative nonfiction writing group told me I should write a memoir about chasing Holden's epilepsy diagnosis, so one day I allowed myself to imagine it. I pinned up five printouts of my defunct blog, poem drafts, bits of essays, and even some fuller essay scenes onto a board in the architecture department. I traced themes across the paper with a yellow highlighter and used Post-It notes to jot down connections. At the end of a four-hour session with myself and my thermos of tea, I had a vision of this book, of my own chaotic "travel"/parenting memoir. After imagining what a memoir might look like, I photographed my collage and called it Draft A.

Writing a book-length memoir was new terrain for me. I composed a long list of important moments that chronicled the early seizures and attempts to find a diagnosis, but for several years, finding my way through the writing occurred in fits and starts. I could only focus on it sporadically in the two years after Xavier was born. I developed the scraps into vignettes, and then received some feedback at a writing conference, which inspired me to keep going. I fleshed out longer scenes, and then hired an expert on motherhood memoirs to respond to my draft. Despite these milestones, and consistently receiving responses from my best friend and my creative nonfiction writing group, I didn't have a complete draft until 2019. I called that Draft F.

Around the same time that Dr. Jones declared Holden "free" of active LKS, I sent Draft F to an editor with an excellent reputation. My hopes were high. I thought I knew where the draft had landed—almost ready for publication. I wanted feedback on sentences to polish and suggestions for possible places to submit it. Her feedback was wise but felt devastating: the chapters read too much like essays. She gave ample comments, but I had to figure out how to revise the layers to create a different structure. I had relied on the kind of composing I already knew, and I had to learn new tactics on my own.

Six weeks after I received this feedback, the COVID-19 pandemic unfolded across the globe, and like so many other millions of people, everything about our day-to-day life changed. Although I heard many stories of people crushed by illness and pandemic chaos, for the most part, Brian and I adapted: we both taught online at home, and I taught Holden and Xavier there, too. After we adjusted to our new day-to-day rhythms, I carved out time to work. I woke up at 5:00 a.m. every morning so I could harness every ounce of concentration. This process didn't feel chaotic or stressful as my intense parenting had felt, but it required a similar willingness to embrace humility, acquire new skills, and submit to trial and error.

* * *

It feels like a strange blend of serendipity and irony that it took moving to a new country to give me a fuller respect for "Welcome to Holland" as well as provide the stories, theories, and strategies I needed. In May 2021, when Holden was fifteen, Brian got a job offer at the University of Manitoba in Winnipeg. A job contract for me followed two months later. The decision to move to Winnipeg felt significant. We decided to think through the possibilities carefully but trust our abilities to work tactically along the way. Brian and I listed all the reasons to move and all the reasons to stay. We acknowledged the risks. I remember thinking, "Do I trust him to have my back if something doesn't work out? Do I trust that his actions and words will align and stay aligned?" I did. So, in July and August 2021, still in the midst of the pandemic, we sold our house, packed up our belongings, and moved to Canada.

I assumed that *Silence and Seizure* would be published shortly after we moved. An editor at a press in the States had been in contact with me, and our meetings via video call had felt encouraging. But just as Brian, Holden, Xavier, and I were moving into our new house, I received some specific feedback: I needed to centre disability more clearly.

There were moments as we settled into our new jobs and lives in Winnipeg that I recognized opportunities presenting themselves, moments where seemingly disparate strands of my life began informing each other more directly. Since I'd joined the Women's and Gender Studies department, not the English department, I'd needed to develop new classes, including a course at the intersection of feminism and disability. I'd begun to research feminist disability studies, a theory new to me, and thus I'd started to find the theories I needed to revise my frameworks yet again.

Researching feminist disability studies for my future course changed the way I saw my manuscript, and frankly, my relationship to disability as Holden's mom. In my self-designed crash course, I read Rosemarie Garland-Thomson's 2005 article "Feminist Disability Studies" and then found her website.[2] Then each night for weeks, I listened to her recorded lectures and others I found as I made dinner. Because she often discusses disability in the context of literature and narratives, her ideas met a ready space in my mind. I was stunned by my own lack of knowledge about the discourse of disability, a lack that echoed my dearth of knowledge about epilepsy after Holden's first seizure. I had so much to learn (and created a to-read book list nearly as long as my comprehensive exam bibliography for my doctoral program), but her work was a catalyst for reflection as I thought about *Silence and Seizure* and my experiences that I represented.

Even though I hadn't engaged it directly in my manuscript at the time, I saw that implicit in the gaps, in the ways I juxtaposed images, and in the places I pointed to a truth in dialogue, that I'd begun to resist the medical model of disability. I'd begun to resist the attitude of defect and I'd begun to question the dominant narratives professionals sought to apply to my son. Before encountering the theory, I'd begun to revise. Learning feminist and critical disability studies theories gave me more concrete language to name and understand the muddled confusion, the ever-pervasive feeling of lack (of knowledge, of experience, of help), and the reason the abyss surfaced for me before Holden's diagnosis. But after I'd become acquainted with theory, I had a decision to make: how should I use it to explicitly shape *Silence and Seizure*?

How many times, being Holden's parent, did I think I finally understood before something shifted and I realized that understanding was only partial, only contextual?

How many times, in writing this book, did I think I finally found the right word, right sentence, right scene before I encountered a new insight that sent me back in to revise?

I decided to thread the theory throughout the narrative and engage it meaningfully. So it followed that just like my parenting took on dimensions I didn't expect, the book did too. I thought I was writing a lyric memoir focused on chasing down my son's diagnosis and surviving several different kinds of loss, but the decision to engage with the theory explicitly provided me with a way to complete the book I needed to write, not that one I intended to write.

I will always be Holden's mother, always learning alongside him and from him, always adding to my breadth and depth of knowledge about my child and myself. I will always be a writer, reflecting on my experiences and thinking about them in new ways. I will always be immersed in the intersections of theory, story, and experience, engaging with tactics for flourishing.

* * *

"So, Holden," I said as he walked through the room while I was working this epilogue. "I'm almost done writing the book where you're a main character." We'd spoken about it before, but not for a few months.

"Cool!" he said.

"I talk about your epilepsy in the book. Is that okay?"

"Yeah. I saw a photo of me during an EEG at the hospital," Holden said. "And there were two photos of me with my dog, Haven."

"In your photobook?" I asked.

"Yeah. Haven was a good dog. She slept next to my bed."

"I remember. She was a good dog. I miss her," I said. She'd died the spring before we moved to Canada. The vet thought she'd had cancer, but it was sudden, even at her age of ten and a half.

"I'd get her up in the morning," Holden said. I nodded. Holden wanted to talk about Haven, a topic he didn't often choose. "I picked out Haven at the store. We took her home from the groomer's." I wondered where Holden got that idea. We'd never shopped for dogs before, or any pet for that matter.

"Not exactly. Remember? You met her once, and you played fetch with her, and then the next time you had an EEG, her trainer brought her to the hospital, and we brought her home."

"Oh, yeah. So I picked her out...." Holden blended our versions. But this time I didn't correct him, I just narrated the details about the day we met Haven for the first time.

I often wonder what details he remembers about his childhood; he rarely offers them when I ask. And except for recalling electrodes, shampooing out sticky glue, and playing the Wii in his hospital room, he doesn't have much to say about his seizure disorder. We mostly talk about his favourite subjects: movies, video games, music, and road trips.

And, these days, many more topics make it into the mix: taekwondo (Holden, Xavier, and I joined our neighbourhood club); our family's epic vacation to Quebec City, Montreal, and Ottawa; Holden's Canadian neurologist declaring his EEG clear. He's been off medication completely for nearly two years. I resist linear narratives of progress and ending with stories that explain "where Holden is now, cognitively" as one reader of an earlier version of this book asked for. Holden's still unfolding, revealing thoughts and nuances in his personality. He's still articulating likes and dislikes that the seizures and medications once obscured. Holden's gifts are many, and he's still discovering them. Holden would say this was "cool," and I'd say that I enjoy all the lovely discoveries unfolding.

ACKNOWLEDGEMENTS

I AM SO GRATEFUL TO EVERYONE WHO CONTRIBUTED TO THE existence of this book. Friends, family, academic colleagues, and members of my writing community supplied a range of support: encouraging words, constructive feedback, time and energy, and financial gifts and grants. In particular, I'd like to thank those who provided formative feedback: Rochelle Harris Cox, Amber Jensen, Mary Woster Haug, Diane Driedger, Ana Maria Spagna, Kate Hopper, Anne Horowitz, James Engelhardt, Shaun Vigil, Sonja Boon, Marlene Kadar, and several anonymous peer reviewers. Thanks also goes out to Lian Reese, who provided assistance early in the submission process, Marianne Zarzana, who created paths for drafts to take shape, and Jocelyn Thorpe, who introduced me to the Life Writing Series at Wilfrid Laurier University Press.

I am fortunate to have support of the University of Manitoba's Faculty of Arts and Faculty of Education as well as my colleagues in Women's and Gender Studies and Disability Studies.

Silence and Seizure would not be possible without the support of my family. My brother, Terrance, and his partner, Kell, were steadfast cheerleaders; my mother read early drafts of the manuscript, and both she and my father offered words of encouragement. Holden's father, Abel, gave me his consent to share these words and always recognized the love for Holden at the heart of this book. Brian believed in the potential of this story from the very beginning and became a fierce protector of my words and my time. Xavier gave me love and inspiration, and Holden—well, this book would not exist without Holden's consistent love and care.

I'm grateful to live on Treaty One in Winnipeg, a place where I learn from the prairies and rivers, from the city and its diversity, and from the Indigenous peoples who have lived here for generations. I value the relationships that being here has encouraged me to engage, and I hope to contribute as a good relative should.

NOTES

PREFACE

1 I've used several resources over the years to learn and to teach the ethics of creative nonfiction, and one of the most common topics covered in these books, articles, and websites is the representation of others. Sondra Perl and Mimi Schwartz address "writing about family" in their classic textbook *Writing True: The Art and Craft of Creative Nonfiction* (158–60) and use the advice of other writers as the bottom line: "Write honestly, but with respect" (158). Brenda Miller and Suzanne Paola emphasize attention to these "tricky issues," yet argue that "it's vital to remember that your story *is* your story to tell" (*Tell It Slant: Writing and Shaping Creative Nonfiction,* 70). The "grandfather of creative nonfiction," Lee Gutkind, includes the chapter "Family Members as Characters" in *Keep It Real: Everything You Need to Know About Researching and Writing Creative Nonfiction*, outlining some of the advantages and disadvantages of doing so and urging readers to "think carefully" (61). This kind of

advice informed the foundation of my approach when I began this book project, especially as I came to appreciate the nuance of my particular context of writing about a disabled family member.

2 Although I've written many persona poems in which the speaker is not a version of me, I tend to treat the "I" point of view in poetry as a version of myself with an allegiance to veracity. Generally, I am open to small shifts of fact and use images that help me achieve emotional truth, but I rarely straight-out *lie*. My mentor, Ted Kooser, influenced this attitude early in my graduate work with him. In "Lying for the Sake of Making Poems," published in *After Confession: Poetry as Autobiography*, Kooser writes: "When 'I' says something happened, I believe it happened, and if something awful has happened to 'I,' I feel for the poet" (159). Many other poets weigh in on issues of "ethical and aesthetic considerations" in this volume, and they shaped my approach too, including Kate Sontag's "Mother, May I? Writing with Love" and Judith Harris's "Breaking the Code of Silence: Ideology and Women's Confessional Poetry."

3 Kate Hopper's *Use Your Words: A Writing Guide for Mothers* helped me think through how to represent my children as characters in my initial foray into *Silence and Seizure*. Hopper urges writers to take care in how readers initially see them—as kids, as people—before introducing their differences: "…so often if we know someone is different, whether it's because this person has a disability or was adopted, we attach a whole set of expectations and stereotypes to him or her, and this gets in the way of actually seeing the person there; we end up only seeing the difference" (52). And yet I needed more. I adapted advice blogs on "writing about your kids" and disabled kids in particular, creating a list of practices that resonated with me. Some tips, such as to stay anonymous and change my name, aren't possible in a book like this. But others, such as to consider the actions I am modelling and becoming aware of disability tropes, I took seriously. What became most important to me was to tell my story, not my child's story. Although I sometimes speculate on what Holden is thinking, and I certainly had to anticipate his needs and wants for several years when he couldn't tell me, I don't pretend to know how he makes meaning from the experiences we've shared.

4 Two essays helped me understand more clearly the conversations I was entering as a writer and a mother of a disabled child. In "Feminist Disability Studies," Rosemarie Garland-Thomson argues that this particular kind of scholarship reimagines disability by "probing the cultural meanings attributed to bodies that societies deem disabled" (1557). Garland-Thomson gave me language for my sense of disability "as a system of exclusions that stigmatizes human differences" (1557). I'd been asked to reimagine disability before reading Garland-Thomson, but I hadn't named the system of exclusions, nor had I interrogated the cultural meanings of disability I was beginning to articulate. The second essay was Alison Piepmeier's "Saints, Sages, and Victims: Endorsement of and Resistance to Cultural Stereotypes in Memoirs by Parents of Children with Disabilities," published in *Disability Studies Quarterly*. Piepmeier criticizes parent memoirs that "reinforce and thereby strengthen our culture's dehumanizing stereotypes that surround and define disability" (par. 1). She argues that they often dehumanize the child and use excessive grief to propel the narrative. Although I'd already attempted to resist these harmful tropes in an early version of this book, after reading her article, I made this resistance more direct.

5 Quinn and Long, "Consent-as-Method: Capacity to Consent of Cognitively Disabled People and Research Ethics Review," 111.

6 Quinn and Long, "Consent-as-Method," 111. This article, published in *Canadian Journal of Disability Studies*, framed the importance of paying attention to the various ways Holden indicated consent, not only with words but also with his gestures and attitude. Quinn and Long explain how they developed "protocols based on participants' existing strategies and practices" (110), which included "expressions, fleeting comments, bodies-in-spaces, and stims, all of which served to express a felt sense of our consenting relations-feeling together" (110). Some of Holden's existing practices included attending to our conversation with his body language, responding to visual images with stories, articulating his emotions, and reflecting.

PROLOGUE

1 In the first entry to *Keywords in Disability Studies*, editors Rachel Adams, Benjamin Reiss, and David Serlin tackle the ever-shifting definition of disability: "Disability encompasses a broad range of bodily, cognitive, and sensory differences and capacities" (5). Historically, people with these differences were described as invalid, crippled, deviant, limited, slow, deformed, mad; disability conferred a stigmatized status (5–7). In recent decades, scholars and activists have pushed back against the framing of disability as defect, advocating for a "positive identity category" (8). In this book, the diverse and sometimes conflicting definitions of disability inform my use of the word, but I generally think of disability as contextual. Disability occurs when a person exists in a world not designed with their body in mind. In the chronological timeline of this memoir, I did not have a nuanced understanding of disability or disability studies—the academic branch that studies the interdisciplinary nature of disability history and culture. And yet my research has since informed the lens through which I now understand and make meaning from this period of my life.

2 The medical model of disability locates the problem of disability in the body of the disabled person, whereas the social model of disability locates the problem in social institutions and environments; it is society that disables a person with its complex sets of exclusions. As Alison Kafer argues: "Once disability has been placed solely in the medical framework, and both disability and the medical world are portrayed as apolitical, then disability has no place in radical politics or social movements—except as a problem to be eradicated" (*Feminist, Queer, Crip*, 9). For much of Holden's childhood, the medical model's emphasis on cure and pathology informed my sense of understanding what was happening in our lives and shaped my decisions. It's not that medical science and medical professionals were unnecessary—they were important elements in helping Holden survive his seizure disorder—but that the values, assumptions, and practices of the medical model precluded other ways of thinking that would have been helpful, perhaps even transformative. Kafer offers a political and relational model, "positioning 'disability' as

a set of practices and associations that can be critiqued, contested, and transformed" (9). I find hers and other models of disability that emphasize fluidity and relationality far more generative and empowering.

3 Ashley Eisenmenger's definition of ableism on the website *Access Living* helped me distill my conceptual understanding of the term, which I think of as discrimination against a person or persons who are disabled or assumed to be. Ableism is often used without definition, similar to the ways other forms of discrimination—such as racism or sexism—are used. Fiona Kumari Campbell describes it as "the ideological hypervaluation of ableness and the ways in which such norms of abled and disabled identity are given force in law, social policy, and cultural values" (13). Campbell's definition emphasizes the effects of valuing certain kinds of bodies over others, which is helpful in criticizing the impact of ableism and advocating for change.

4 In an interview with Alison Kafer, Nirmala Erevelles argues, "The humanities-oriented focus on disability as transgressive text is extremely effective in deconstructing normativity but often does very little to explain how—quite literally—to survive in an ableist world" (207). Survival in an ableist world became a touchstone in my reflections about my parenting. Erevelles's work persuaded me that any analysis of disability should be relational and situated within historical, material, and structural contexts and conditions. I've tried to situate my story within the contexts and conditions that felt most salient: the privileges of my race and education level, for example, and the disadvantages of living in a rural town without access to the medical and support resources we needed.

CHAPTER ONE

1 Early in my role as Assistant Professor at South Dakota State University, my department head tasked me with growing the creative writing curriculum. One way I did this was by creating a course that satisfied the second-year writing objectives and centred particular kinds of research practices. While still a graduate student, I published a chapbook of poetry

inspired by the life of Catherine of Siena (*The Love of Unreal Things*). My inquiry into the scholarship of Catherine's life guided my writing, so I used aspects of my process as a model for this course design. In addition to Lee Ann Roripaugh's *Year of the Snake* and Margaret Atwood's *The Journals of Susanna Moodie*, other books shaped my decision-making as well: *Becoming Bone: Poems on the Life of Celia Thaxter (1836–1894)* by Annie Boutelle and *Lizzie Borden in Love: Poems in Women's Voices* by Julianna Baggott. In Introduction to Creative Writing, my students visited museum archives for the research that informed their poems.

2 The thread of writing practice that I introduce in this chapter can be traced to the influence of Zora Neale Hurston's *Dust Tracks on a Road: An Autobiography*, Audre Lorde's *Zami: A New Spelling of My Name: A Biomythography*, and Maya Angelou's *I Know Why the Caged Bird Sings*. Writing framed my initial readings of these books: I knew each of these writers first as a novelist or poet, so reading about their lives and what shaped their sensibilities as writers made a deep impact. Although I've read dozens of memoirs since reading these three, teaching them over the years has strengthened my admiration of these works. And because my writing practice shaped my parenting practice (and vice versa), I found it an important touchstone to include in my own memoir.

3 About 50 million people worldwide have epilepsy (World Health Organization, 2024), but despite its prevalence as a common neurological disorder, myths persist regarding what seizures look like, what happens during a seizure, and how to respond. Seizures can be caused by high fevers, brain infections, serious illness, lack of sleep, low blood sodium levels, and brain injuries (Mayo Clinic, "Seizures," 2024). What a seizure looks like can include "short-lived confusion, a staring spell, jerking movements of the arms and legs… loss of consciousness or awareness, changes in thinking or emotions" (Mayo Clinic, "Seizures," 2024). Basic first-aid response calls for staying with the person, removing anything near them that could cause injury, turning the person onto their left side with their mouth pointing toward the ground, and timing the seizure; if it lasts more than five minutes, emergency services should be called (Centers for Disease Control and Prevention).

CHAPTER TWO

1 Denise Grady, "Doctors Put Hope in Thin Wires to Ease the Clutches of Epilepsy," A20, pars. 12–13.

2 See Grady A20, par. 6.

3 Because medical professionals aren't usually around to observe a seizure, diagnosis can be tricky, so neurologists combine a patient's detailed medical history with brain imaging. A routine electroencephalogram (EEG) is usually indicated first, which typically happens at an outpatient clinic for a few hours. If a neurologist reads the data produced by the test and sees abnormal brain activity, they can often figure out the type of seizures the patient is having and create a treatment plan (Johns Hopkins Medicine, "Diagnosing Seizures and Epilepsy").

4 The Epilepsy Foundation, a nonprofit organization, publishes Epilepsy.com. The mission of this organization is to "promote education, policy, research, and systemic change that will foster measurable and sustainable improvement for all people living with epilepsy" (Epilepsy Foundation, "About the Foundation"). Although the information on Epilepsy.com has been revised since my early research quests, these statistics can still be found there. Editors have replaced the "Epilepsy 101" tab with an alternative (and more descriptive) organization: Understanding Seizures, Seizure Triggers, Types of Seizures, Epilepsy Syndromes, Facts and Statistics about Epilepsy, Causes of Epilepsy, Diagnosis, Treatment, Complications and Risks. The website editors also introduce jargon and define acronyms more effectively than I remember on earlier versions of the website.

5 Types of seizures, or how medical professionals describe and classify seizures, are complex and evolving. In 2017, seven years after our appointment with Helen, there was another change in terminology—even beyond the changes she described. In this book, I try to convey how my actual learning about seizures unfolded, but I want to note that better education tools are now available than those I found in 2010. My recent foray into the internet revealed many websites with dated terminology, but the Epilepsy Foundation has one of the most accessible websites to learn about seizure types, including written articles

and videos with closed captioning. I found it a bit ironic that the first argument epilepsy specialist Dr. Orrin Devinsky makes in the video "Types of Seizures" is that understanding different seizure types is "very, very important," because "what type of seizure has great implications for activities of daily life"; it took years for me to learn how Holden's seizures would affect his daily life. Generally, factors that affect how types of seizures are identified depend on when a seizure begins, a person's level of awareness during a seizure, and whether physical movements happen during a seizure.

6 For years, my interactions with the medical professionals associated with epilepsy at this hospital inspired anger; I could only focus on what they had done wrong and what they did awkwardly. I was also mad at myself for not being a better advocate for Holden and for not asking for a second opinion sooner. Reading Jillian Horton's memoir *We Are All Perfectly Fine: A Memoir of Love, Medicine, and Healing* helped me resolve this anger. Horton is a medical doctor whose career was inspired by her sister Wendy, "a martini of a human you could never mix again" (7). Wendy had profound disabilities caused, in part, by how doctors had "screwed up" her case. Horton's experience with a disabled family member strengthened her ethos, but it was her deep, honest, and reflective practice in the pages of the memoir that persuaded me to see doctors differently. The book focuses on Horton's reluctant journey to create a different style of being a doctor—one that embraces mindfulness, authenticity, and the wholeness of being human.

7 *Epilepsia*, the "official journal of the International League Against Epilepsy," published an article about the kindling model on June 1, 2007. "The Relevance of Kindling for Human Epilepsy" describes kindling as "the process by which repeatedly induced seizures result in an increasing seizure duration and enhanced behavioural involvement of those induced seizures until a plateau is reached" (Bertram, 66). Edward Bertram, the article's author, explains the historical development of this tool, what it has revealed about epilepsy, and its limitations for human applications.

8 Morales, *Kindling: Writings on the Body* (Palabrera, 2013), 35.

9 Morales, *Kindling*, 10.

10 Many websites explain seizure thresholds and what can trigger a seizure. The Epilepsy Foundation's "Seizure Triggers" lists and explains commonly reported triggers, describes how to tell whether something is a trigger, and defines "reflex epilepsy"—when seizures are a response to very specific situations.

11 Morales, *Kindling*, 87.

CHAPTER THREE

1 I read the ubiquitous *What to Expect When You're Expecting* when I was pregnant with Holden. The book emphasizes behaviour changes to reduce the risks of miscarriage and premature birth and to increase the chances of a healthy pregnancy. Many readers of this book—and of similar books, websites, and resources—note that one consequence can be an overwhelming preoccupation with the "right behaviour." If something worrisome pops up during the pregnancy or after the baby's birth, the mother may blame herself or others may blame her. Heather Lanier's *Raising a Rare Girl* opens with an amusing catalogue of all the things she did and avoided to "make a SuperBaby." Lanier notes: "Of course, I followed the medical advice standard for women of my generation" (8). Even for women like us who appreciated a good to-do list, the most meticulous planning didn't mean our fertility, childbirth, or children would turn out as planned. Neither Lanier nor I, for example, expected to raise children with rare health conditions.

2 According to a website published by the United Kingdom's Miscarriage Association, a missed or silent miscarriage "is one where the baby has died or not developed, but has not been physically miscarried." Often, there are no physical signs, such as pain or bleeding, to indicate the death of the fetus. There's no consensus in the medical community that explains the delay between the death of the fetus and the scan that diagnoses the miscarriage. Due to pregnancy hormones, the mother often still feels pregnant (The Miscarriage Association, "Missed Miscarriage").

3 This statistic was published by the American College of Obstetricians and Gynecologists: "Recurrent pregnancy loss is a common clinical

problem in reproduction, occurring in approximately 1 percent of reproductive-aged women. A definite cause is established in no more than 50 percent of couples, and several alleged causes of recurrent pregnancy loss are controversial" (American College of Obstetricians and Gynecologists).

4 Rosemarie Garland-Thomson, "Becoming Disabled," *New York Times*, August 19, 2016, par. 15.

5 Alison Reiheld, "The Event That Was Nothing: Miscarriage as a Liminal Event," *Journal of Social Philosophy* 46, no. 1 (2015): 9–10.

6 Rosemarie Garland-Thomson, "Feminist Disability Studies," *Signs: Journal of Women in Culture and Society* 30, no. 2 (2005): 1558.

7 Heather Love, "Stigma," in *Keywords for Disability Studies*, ed. Rachel Adams, Benjamin Reiss, and David Serlin (New York University Press, 2015), 173–76. Love writes: "Stigma is part of the complex of factors that transform impairment into disability. The term refers to the disapproval and disadvantage that attach to people who are seen as different; its repercussions can be far-reaching. Stigma affects employment, social recognition, educational opportunities, friendship and sex, housing, and freedom from violence" (173).

8 This quotation is taken from the synopsis of the book on promotional websites, such as Amazon. Because I returned this book to the library, I wrote this section in *Silence and Seizure* from my personal notes and memory without verifying my recall because the notes and remembered details motivated me to act. Although I'm confident in my general read of the book, I'm less so regarding the exact statistics.

9 Talking about my experiences with recurrent miscarriage, listening to the stories of other women, and reading scholarly discussions of the subject has taught me a lot, but one lesson stands out: each individual needs the space to articulate their experience, and the language they use to do so should be honoured. I understand why people, including medical professionals, use "baby," but for me that word conjured images of newborns—soft-skinned and milk-scented, their rolls of baby fat swaddled by a blanket, tufts of hair sticking up. That wasn't the product of conception that exited my body in four first-trimester miscarriages, and for me to process the grief and move toward a healthy relationship

with these events, I had to claim the paradox: they weren't babies, but I loved them nonetheless.

CHAPTER FOUR

1 Laurel Richardson, "Writing: A Method of Inquiry," in *Handbook of Qualitative Research*, 2nd ed., edited by Norman K. Denzin and Yvonna S. Lincoln (Sage Publications, 2000), 923.

2 Many writer-scholars have helped me articulate writing as a method of inquiry and self-understanding, including Louise DeSalvo's *Writing as a Way of Healing: How Telling Our Stories Transforms Our Lives*.

3 Tanya Titchkosky, *"Normal,"* in *Keywords for Disability Studies*, ed. Rachel Adams, Benjamin Reiss, and David Serlin (New York University Press, 2015), 131. Titchkosky argues that the meaning of normal has changed across time and context; in medical literature specifically, the commitment to seek normal is relatively new. When I read this book, a decade after Holden's odd behaviour began, I was most stuck by Titchkosky's explanation about the social effort to treat norms as static and "measure how others appear to depart from them" (130) because I'd engaged that way of thinking across my life. Although I'd already begun to honour Holden's learning and development as his own, Titchkosky's work gave me a clear framework for the power of normal as a rigid, often coercive ideology. Engaging disability studies scholarship often clarified my experiences and decisions while at the same time connecting them to social systems and ideologies.

4 Titchkosky, *"Normal,"* 131.

5 Reading memoirs by writers who articulate their experiences as disabled, I've probed the ways they describe their parents' attitudes toward their disability for insight. There's often some sort of liminality described. In Stephen Kuusisto's *Planet of the Blind* (Delta Press, 1998), for example, his vision loss makes him legally blind, "a confusing phrase that means that I can see fractionally, though not enough to truly see" (13); this in-between space creates a "puzzle" for his parents. His mother asserts that he should live like other children, for example, and enrols

him in public school without support. Her attitude seems to shift over time. This work gave more weight to my understanding that even the kinds of disability I imagined as rigidly defined aren't so much. Kuusisto also writes that his parents didn't have resources; there were no "books about blind children or how to bring them up, no associations of parents or support materials" (13). Without ways to help parents rethink "normal," they have a harder time supporting their children to move through a world that disables them.

6 Called *Depakote* in the United States and *Alti-Valproic* in Canada, Divalproex sodium is an anti-epilepsy drug used to stop seizures. It can also be used to treat the manic phase of bipolar disorder and prevent migraines. The Mayo Clinic's description of precautions and side effects is quite extensive; I list just a few in this book.

7 Although medical professionals have an understanding of what happens to neurons during a seizure, it's not always clear what causes neurons to begin errant firing. Seizures can be called *epilepsy* when a person has "two or more seizures at least 24 hours apart that don't have a known cause" (Mayo Clinic, "Seizures"). In about half of the people with epilepsy, no cause can be found, but in the other half, it can be traced to genetics, head trauma, tumours and malformations in the brain, infections, injury before birth, and developmental conditions (Mayo Clinic, "Epilepsy / causes"). As previously noted, changes in the environment or body can lower seizure thresholds and trigger a seizure, but without clear observations by an adult caregiver, it's difficult to trace these patterns in children, if they exist at all. For me this made seizures appear random, and I wondered why Dr. Porter didn't try to ascertain a better understanding of Holden's seizures from the beginning, since no patterns appeared.

8 Although I took notes from this talk, I looked up the definition of SUDEP and statistics about it while composing this scene to verify my notes and memory. The Epilepsy Foundation has a tab on "Early Death and SUDEP" on their website under "Complications and Risks."

CHAPTER FIVE

1 Kristin L. Szuhany and Naomi M. Simon, "Anxiety Disorders: A Review," *JAMA* 328, no. 24 (2022): 2431–45, describe three kinds of anxiety disorder diagnoses: generalized anxiety disorder, social anxiety disorder, and panic disorder; high-functioning anxiety (HFA) isn't among them. It seems to be a culturally created phrase. Lalitaa Suglani notes that HFA "is not currently a recognized anxiety disorder. While it's argued that this is because sufferers tend to function reasonably well in their daily lives, the effects of HFA can be extreme, affecting quality of life and causing intense feelings of loneliness and disconnection" (*High-Functioning Anxiety: A Five-Step Guide to Calming the Inner Panic and Thriving* (Hay House, 2024, xii–xiii). I appreciate this distinction. Not having an official place in the medical literature only emphasizes the point that feeling overwhelmingly anxious is heavily contextual and its tendency to wax and wane depends on other factors in one's life, making it a challenge to identify, trace, and confront.

2 Jillian Lauren's *Everything You Ever Wanted* (Plume Press, 2014) chronicles her journey to adopt her son, Tariku. Early in the book she writes, "As a child, I grew up thinking that adoption was a badge of honor" (44). This comment resonated with me deeply. When her husband, Scott, has a few reservations at the beginning, I saw echoes of my experience with Abel, which also aligned with stories friends had shared about the adoption process; their partners always seemed hesitant at first, then assented to the plan. Later in the book, when Lauren struggles to find explanations for Tariku's aggressive behaviour and resources for support, I recognized my own impulses to cast a net of research and sort through it. This book, as well as other parent memoirs, helped me connect the threads of my experiences with the cultural tapestries we're co-creating as members of society.

3 It's a challenge to write about divorce and to honour the feelings as I once had, especially after they've changed. Abel is a particularly tough character to represent because this book centres the end of our marriage—excluding our years of happiness—and it doesn't attempt to include his perspective. In many ways, it reduces a complex relationship

to a few scenes. Before I began submitting this memoir for publication (an earlier version of this book), I sent him a draft and asked him for his response. He wrote, "This is your story, and it should be told as you experienced it." I value this affirmation, and his appreciation regarding how the book reveals my love for our son.

4 Chloe Jones and Colin Reilly, "Parental Anxiety in Childhood Epilepsy: A Systematic Review," *Epilepsia* 57, no. 4 (2016): 529.

5 Aynur Pekcanlar Akay et al., "Maternal Reactions to a Child with Epilepsy: Depression, Anxiety, Parental Attitudes and Family Functions," *Epilepsy Research* 95, no. 3 (2011): 213–20. See in particular "Results."

6 R. Lv, L. Wu, et al., "Depression, Anxiety and Quality of Life in Parents of Children with Epilepsy," *Acta Neurologica Scandinavica* 120 (2009): 335.

7 Lynn Chapieski et al., "Adaptive Functioning in Children with Seizures: Impact of Maternal Anxiety about Epilepsy," *Epilepsy & Behavior* 7, no. 2 (2005): 246–52. See in particular "Introduction."

8 Joanne Limburg's *Letters to My Weird Sisters: On Autism and Feminism* helped me think more about the dissatisfaction I felt when reading these studies on anxiety in the parents of children with epilepsy. She recounts the blame that early researchers of autism attributed to the mothers of autistic children and defends these mothers, who were most likely doing their best to nurture and raise their children ("Letter to Frau V"). The studies seem to criticize anxious mothers for making their children's lives worse. Limburg also discusses the "good neoliberal Autism Mother," who "willingly takes on the burden of ensuring her child's well-being, which she does in a resilient, independent and entrepreneurial fashion," but argues that mothers shouldn't have to do this kind of work (178). She points to the common occurrence of social services failing to support parents and their disabled children. In doing so, Limburg uses the social model of disability framework to remind readers that it is the responsibility of society to remove the barriers that disable families.

9 Akay et al., "Depression, Anxiety and Quality of Life," discussion, par. 2.

CHAPTER SIX

1 Considering all the available tools to support children with different neurotypes is important, so I don't wish to overly criticize websites like CHADD. Often what brings parents to these websites is worry, and parents use the medical model framing for ADHD pervasive in North America. I believe that critically engaging these kinds of resources is important, though, because often our framing affects the ways parents advocate. If such a high percentage of children present with ADHD, why don't parents pressure schools to provide more support and different ways of engaging these students?

2 CHADD, "For Parents and Caregivers," par. 1.

3 Using neuroimaging to understand ADHD is an evolving field in neurobiology. On several websites about ADHD, I saw the assertion of imaging studies showing differences, so I read the article "Neuroimaging in Attention-Deficit/Hyperactivity Disorder" to learn more. Its authors, Victor Pereira-Sanchez and Francisco X. Castellanos, analyzed forty studies published between January 2019 and September 2020 reporting or reviewing MRI research on ADHD. One consortium "has identified statistically robust, albeit small, differences in structural brain cortical and subcortical indices in children with ADHD versus typically developing controls" (105). Despite this, they ultimately argue that "Neuroimaging in ADHD is still far from informing clinical practice" (105). It seems that pointing to this neurobiological difference isn't yet useful at the individual level, but I think it can help us understand it more generally.

4 Access to education is a common theme in the parent memoirs I've read. The last chapter in Heather Lanier's *Raising a Rare Girl* portrays Fiona's first day at a public kindergarten, a major win for Lanier and her husband. Jillian Lauren's *Everything You Ever Wanted* chronicles Jillian and Scott's foray into finding a preschool that can accommodate Tariku's needs; as a child traumatized by his time spent in an orphanage before his adoption, Tariku acts from a place of fear. In *My Heart Can't Even Believe It*, Amy Silverman represents the tensions around enrolling her daughter, Sophie, in a kindergarten in Arizona:

"...the preschool administrators had been so encouraging about Sophie, telling me she was one of the smartest kids with Down syndrome they'd ever seen.... Yet they had no intention of mainstreaming her at our home school with her sister. Instead, they wanted her in a self-contained classroom at another school" (158). In *Raising Henry: A Memoir of Motherhood, Disability, and Discovery*, Rachel Adams portrays her worry that her son Henry won't get a spot in her New York neighbourhood's Bank Street Family Centre, celebrated for its "integrated program where disabled and nondisabled children attended class together" (147). In each of these books, parents invest hours of work (research, interviews, applications, and networking with other parents, for example) to find places where their children can receive the support and services they need to maximize their education. This level of advocacy speaks to the ways disabled children and their families are not served equally by public institutions and systems. Although I include only a few scenes of my experiences as Holden's educational advocate in this book, I can relate to the level of mental and emotional investment I expended to try to make sure that Holden was taught in places that put his flourishing first.

5 As I wrote and revised this book, I confronted my lack of knowledge about *cognition* despite my obsession with *learning*. Ralph James Savarese's essay "Cognition" introduced me to concepts such as *embodied cognition* and *embedded cognition* that I'm eager to think more about outside the scope of *Silence and Seizure*. Savarese writes: "*Embodied cognition* repairs the traditional mind–body divide, whereas *embedded cognition* reveals the extent to which we all depend on our physical and social environments to think. The former thus blurs the line between 'physical' and 'mental' disabilities because no condition is strictly one or the other, and the latter points to complex accommodative ecologies that enhance cognition by imaginatively distributing it beyond the individual" (40). These concepts help me continue to unsettle the bodymind binary and consider the ways in which Holden's sensory input may have shaped his cognition. It also compels me to think of his "ecologies" of learning and communication.

CHAPTER SEVEN

1 Solomon describes his capacious theory of identity in "Son." Each subsequent chapter in *Far from the Tree* illuminates Solomon's argument in specific ways by providing evidence from case studies he has conducted and families he has interviewed. He includes groups of disabled people united by diagnosis, with chapter titles such as "Dwarfs," "Down Syndrome," "Autism," and "Schizophrenia," as well as nondisabled groups united by their relationship to a stigmatized status, such as "Rape" and "Crime." I was most interested in Solomon's focus on family units and how parents negotiate their relationships with children they don't perceive as much like themselves.

2 Andrew Solomon, *Far from the Tree: Parents, Children and the Search for Identity* (Scribner Classics, 2014), 2.

3 Solomon, *Far from the* Tree, 2.

4 Solomon, *Far from the Tree,* 4.

5 I don't recall which version of Helen Keller's biography I read as a child, as Keller wrote many herself and many scholars have written about her life, too. I appreciate, however, Georgina Kleege's *Blind Rage: Letters to Helen Keller*, which inspired me to rethink and complicate the version of Keller I'd learned about as a child. *Blind Rage* recreates imagined conversations that Kleege has with Keller, at once an icon and a "personal demon" (ix). The series of letters "invites the reader to inhabit Keller's consciousness" in a way that allows Kleege to explore her "shared experiences and sensibilities" (x) with Keller.

6 I read Emily Rapp's *The Still Point of a Turning World* five years after that day in Manchester when I imagined disappearing, so when I read her words, "Everything in me wanted to look away, to disappear, and often, to die" (48), they resonated deeply. Rapp's journey of parenting a disabled child is radically different from mine, however, as she learned of her son's diagnosis with the fatal Tay-Sachs disease when he was only a few months old. The depth of her grief and the articulation of her need to make meaning became an exquisitely painful touchstone for me: "I wanted to be present for my son, but my mind needed to spin and spin and spin, searching for solutions, the salve of meaning, story, language.

Instead, I only generated more questions, a kind of frantic curiosity that would, for a brief moment, stave off the feelings of helplessness and rage, the gripping, shattering, closing-in sadness like two hands rattling the heart" (47–48). Reading how she coped with and survived the death of her son illustrated how courage can be a choice.

7 Solomon, *Far from the Tree*, 6.

8 Solomon, *Far from the Tree*, 6.

9 Since the writing of this chapter, Epilepsy.com has changed its description of epilepsy syndromes—although it still lists the types and symptoms in similar ways. The two that seemed to describe Holden the best, but that I disregarded, have combined under a new name: Developmental Epileptic Encephalopathy with Spike Wave Activation in Sleep, DEE-SWAS. See more in the chapter nine notes.

10 Solomon, *Far from the Tree*, 5.

11 Solomon, *Far from the Tree*, 5. Solomon isn't the only scholar who pushes against unhelpful dichotomies such as illness and identity to help us understand our relationship to disability. In *Brilliant Imperfection*, Eli Clare explores the contradictions of cure, the "deeply held belief that body–minds considered broken need to be fixed. Cure serves many purposes. It saves lives, manipulates lives, and prioritizes some lives over others" (cover). Specifically, Clare asks us to reconsider normal/abnormal and natural/unnatural: "Can a body–mind be deemed both natural and abnormal? And when are those moments and locations of disability and chronic pain unnatural—as unnatural as war, toxic landfills, childhood abuse, and poverty?" (53). By grappling with complications of cure throughout the book, he points our attention to specific contexts where the binaries collapse without diminishing human experience.

12 Solomon, *Far from the Tree*, 5.

CHAPTER EIGHT

1 Brian explained palimpsest from his accumulated professional knowledge, but when I asked to learn more, he showed me the work of Bernard Tschumi. For a richer discussion of the palimpsest as a

principle of architectural design, see Tschumi's collection of essays, *Architecture and Disjunction* (MIT Press, 1996). The first page of "Abstract Mediation and Strategy" opens with Tschumi outlining urbanistic program design options for an architect, including composition, complement, palimpsest, and mediation (191–92).

2 When I composed this chapter, I reread Brian's emails, which I had saved. I paraphrased or quoted him from this period of personal correspondence with his explicit permission.

3 The judgments of others regarding parenting may be universally perceived, but for parents of children with disabilities, public scrutiny can be particularly painful. The tacit criticism I sensed from the other women in the salon that day unnerved me; I felt watched and judged the whole time, because many people who don't have experiences with disabled children blame parents for any "bad" behaviour. In the parenting memoirs and essays I've read, parents are often accused of everything from not caring enough to caring too much, from being too permissive to not permissive enough. Sometimes they are even criticized for bringing their children to public spaces. Similarly, the children are often labelled "bad" or "disruptive." Even professionals who work with disabled children develop their own narratives.

Caryn Mirriam-Goldberg's essay "Dragonflies and Inky Blackness: Raising a Child with Asperger's Syndrome" captures the range of viewpoints that can be assigned to one child: "To kids his own age he's a nuisance. To the school district he's a special needs child. To psychologists he's a quandary. To teachers he's a challenge. To relatives he's a little too hyper. To other parents, he's annoying. To piles of paperwork he's another diagnosis of Asperger's syndrome, epilepsy, hyperactivity. To child-rearing books he's an exception to the rule" (242). Understanding that it wasn't only my parenting strategies being judged, but also my child, made public episodes like what happened in the salon even more difficult to experience.

4 Many of the poems I composed that summer were included in *The Poet & The Architect*. Inspired by my relationship with Brian, this book of poetry explores family-making and place-making using architectural imagery and metaphor.

CHAPTER NINE

1 Porochista Khakpour's *Sick: A Memoir* is a journey of failed diagnoses and faltering relationships, themes that I drew on when composing *Silence and Seizure*. These twin trajectories—Khakpour's quest for physical health and healthy relationships—generate tension, ushering readers into the complexity of her life. As she negotiates her career as a writer and academic, moving from place to place for different opportunities (New York; Santa Fe; Los Angeles; Maryland; Pennsylvania; Illinois), she frames herself as somewhat nomadic yet always embodied, simultaneously walking the boundaries of wellness and addiction. Honest and introspective yet equally critical of the social forces that circumscribe our health, Khakpour reveals a complex life shaped by disease.

2 In 2022, the International League Against Epilepsy (ILAE) changed the classification of epilepsy syndromes (Manokaran, Sharma, and Ramachandrannair). These changes help articulate the differences between epilepsy and encephalopathy, the latter of which is a "pronounced brain dysfunction affecting mental status and cognitive processes" (Sands and Gelinas, 24), especially in regard to the development of children who have an epileptic encephalopathy—brain dysfunction caused by seizure activity. In an article appearing in *Pediatric Neurology*, Sands and Gelinas describe the complexity of Developmental or Epileptic Encephalopathy with Spike-Wave Activation in Sleep (DEE-SWAS). Previously referred to as ESES (encephalopathy related to electrographic status epilepticus during slow sleep), or CSWS (continuous spike-and-wave in sleep), DEE-SWAS "is a spectrum of disorders." Landau-Kleffner Syndrome (LKS) is a subtype. Sands and Gelinas describe the challenges of diagnosing and treating DEE-SWAS: "There is no consensus on the electrographic criteria for SWAS (what abundance of spikes are necessary for the diagnosis) … The field is further challenged by the lack of consensus on how to quantify spikes on EEG, by inconsistent assessment of cognitive and behavioural symptoms, and by clinical heterogeneity across affected individuals" (26). This new research puts the experience of our struggle with diagnosis and treatment within a larger medical context and explains that the problems

stemmed from a field-wide lack of understanding, not merely the ignorance of a few experts. It also furthers my conviction that grappling with this kind of epilepsy syndrome requires drawing on research from both the medical sciences and social models of disability to help a child (and adult survivor) flourish.

3 For medical evidence regarding multiple subpial transection, I read a co-authored article published in *Brain* by Christopher L. Grote, Patricia Van Slyke, and Jo-Ann B. Hoeppner. The writers argue that, since there were so few children in the study, it was difficult to generalize the results—but that MST "may be useful in allowing for a restoration of speech and language abilities in children diagnosed with Landau-Kleffner syndrome" (561).

4 Eva Kittay, *Learning from My Daughter: The Value and Care of Disabled Minds* (Oxford: Oxford University Press, 2019), 26–27. *Learning from My Daughter* was an instrumental book in helping me find language for my experiences as Holden's parent. Her discussion of the desire of normalcy in "The New Normal and a Good Life" felt affirming to me, even though I didn't experience the "shock" of the news of abnormality as she did with her daughter's diagnosis. My understanding happened gradually. Furthermore, her questions about grief assisted me with articulating its nuances.

5 When I tried to retrace some of this early internet research more than five years after Holden's LKS diagnosis, the websites had changed. I did find sources that I'd accessed with my university credentials—mostly medical research articles. Michael C. Smith and Thomas J. Hoeppner's "Epileptic Encephalopathy of Late Childhood," published in the *Journal of Clinical Neurophysiology*, explains the historical background of the diagnosis and supplies keywords for understanding the disorder, such as "acquired aphasia," the phrase Drs. Landau and Kleffner used ("Historical Background" and "Nosology"). It also traces some of the terms challenged over the years, including verbal agnosia as opposed to auditory agnosia. The rare occurrence of DEE-SWAS is one of the reasons for these changes. In their 2008 article, "The Landau-Kleffner Syndrome and Epilepsy with Continuous Spike-Waves During Sleep," James J. Riviello, Jr. and Stavros Hadjiloizou supply a statistic: "In a

recent 20-year epidemiologic study of childhood epilepsy, Kramer and colleagues reported LKS and CSWS in 0.2 percent each" (378). Nearly twenty years later, the statistic has changed a bit. Epilepsy.com reports that it affects 1 out of 2,000 (0.5 percent) of children with epilepsy (Joshi, "DEE/SWAS"). Despite an increase in diagnosis, this epilepsy syndrome is still rare.

6 Authors of medical journal articles often mentioned symptoms of language regression but rarely defined or explained terms such as mutism, echolalia, etc. To follow up, I found the work of speech pathologist Carol Sober Alpern, who had conducted research on speech in children with LKS. In "Identification and Treatment of Landau-Kleffner Syndrome," Alpern reviews the literature on LKS with a focus on language regression: "Typically, children show a gradual regression in expressive language. The literature highlights a variety of expressive deficits, including reduced syntactic complexity, telegraphic speech, word-finding deficits, jargon, neologisms, paraphasias, perseveration, and mutism" ("Communication Function"). When I found this list and explored the definitions of these words, I was able to identify the particular symptoms that Holden's speech patterns revealed.

7 I found this explanation in a variety of sources, always attributing it to Drs. Landau and Kleffner. For example, in the article "Epileptic Encephalopathy Syndromes in Infancy," Raidah Albaradie includes this quote in the section "Pathophysiology." I wrote it down in my early parent-driven note-taking, without reference.

8 I am not sure what website defined this word for me, but these were notes I took by hand while doing informal research after Holden's diagnosis. I want to retain this definition since I argue with it later in this chapter.

9 This quotation comes from the neuropsychological report written for the Minnesota Epilepsy Group, dated September 19, 2012 and September 20, 2012.

10 Kittay, *Learning from My Daughter*, 93. Kittay describes disability as a relational trait in the chapter titled "The Ethics of Prenatal Testing and Selection." When I read these words a decade after Holden's diagnosis with LKS, they affirmed my own "working definition" of disability—the way I defined it to myself.

11 Kittay, *Learning from My Daughter*, 115. In "How Not to Argue for Selective Reproductive Procedures," I saw a rough description of what I'd been doing when Kittay argues that "Disability can involve a reorientation toward life that can be neutral or positive" (115). In these ways, the theories and narratives of other mothers and scholars gave me confidence in the ways I'd started making meaning from my experience.

12 See Kittay, *Learning from My Daughter*, especially Chapter Eight, "The Completion of Care—The Normativity of Care." Here Kittay argues for care as a mode of moral conduct (167). Her tripartite "ethics of care" (171) explained the philosophical underpinnings of the labour of mothering and highlighted aspects of dependency and independency I'd never considered. Kittay argues for a relationship between the care-givers and person receiving care grounded in attentive responsiveness made possible "by an empathetic connection to and understanding of the other. These enable us to 'read' the mind of another, especially in cases where the other is either temporarily or permanently incapable of communication through speech. As such, these affective connections are a needed moral epistemic resource" (175). Because I'd seen myself strengthen my own attentive responsiveness in relationship to Holden across time, Kittay's argument bolstered my belief in the importance of this labour. It also turned my attention to the ways I needed to fore-ground Holden's "flourishing" (176), even when it might be hard for me to do so. In my own reflection, I used Kittay's arguments to both clarify and complicate my perspective; this reflection became an essential element to completing *Silence and Seizure*.

13 I also write about the moment of breastfeeding Holden after his birth in my essay "Beyond Sound," published in my book *Chrysopoeia: Essays of Language, Love, and Place*. A few scenes in *Silence and Seizure* have similar, parallel moments in the following essays, also published in *Chrysopoeia:* "Filaments of Prayer," "Once Upon a Tower," and "Disordered." In early versions of this book, I borrowed whole scenes and sections from these essays, but as the revision processes unfolded, I revised them extensively. *Silence and Seizure* offers the experiences in an altered form and from a different perspective, even if one can trace them to their earlier incarnations.

CHAPTER TEN

1 A different context for thinking through disability helped me put my own feelings about how others perceived me into a new and healthier perspective. When I read Audre Lorde's *The Cancer Journals*, I was struck by the receptionist at the doctor's office insisting that Lorde wear a prosthesis because otherwise it was bad "for the morale of the office" (32). Lorde didn't want to wear it and felt confident in herself and in her choice, but the receptionist demanded that Lorde rethink that so she and other healthy individuals in the office would simply feel better. It seemed they didn't want to be reminded of the physical difference that breast cancer can create and held Lorde responsible for sustaining that illusion. Likewise, I felt pressure to ensure that other people weren't disturbed by Holden's behaviour; I felt compelled to sustain their illusion of normalcy in the public space of the mall. Lorde's work helped me understand that it's not my responsibility to make others feel better about my differences or my child's difference.

2 I stumbled upon Susannah Cahalan's *Brain on Fire: My Month of Madness* ten years after Holden's meltdown in the mall, and I regretted not finding it earlier. Cahalan, a journalist, chronicles her experience "falling into madness" due to NMDA-receptor autoimmune encephalitis. In just a month, the twenty-four-year-old went from developing an ambitious writing career and renting her own apartment in New York City to being labelled violent and psychotic. Much of what Cahalan describes gave me insight into what Holden could have experienced but didn't have the words for, including aggression and impulsivity. She also grapples with echolalia and mutism. Cahalan describes the experience of seizures, EEGs, and other medical procedures that Holden submitted to as well. Medical doctors repeatedly misdiagnosed her before one discovered the reason for her symptoms: the right side of her brain was inflamed; it was a rare, newly discovered autoimmune disease. After her doctor found the right course of treatment, it took months for her brain to recover. Reading *Brain on Fire* gave me the insight Holden couldn't describe regarding memory loss, intermittent lucidness, and cognitive recovery. Because I'm writing about what I've observed, I can't articulate

such a complex, embodied reality—but Cahalan does, and I'm grateful for her perspective.

3 In particular, I'm thinking of Chris Gabbard's book, *A Life Beyond Reason: A Father's Memoir*, which traces his experience of fatherhood from the traumatic birth of his first child, August, to August's death fourteen years later. As the book unfolds, Gabbard confronts the significant medical costs and the demands of time and energy for therapies—and yet these barriers don't keep him from advocacy. Gabbard writes, "As August grew older, we grew too. We were learning the difference between disability and impairment" (96). What follows is a discussion of various disability scholars and activists who gave him language for the social model of disability. He engages these conversations not only as a father of a disabled child, but also as a scholar of the Enlightenment. Much of the internal tension in this book arises from the spiritual changes Gabbard undergoes as an atheist. Although subtle, the transformation gives him a way to grapple with August's death and understand the philosophical significance of his relationship to his son.

4 Susannah B. Mintz, "Invisibility," in *Keywords for Disability Studies*, ed. Rachel Adams, Benjamin Reiss, and David Serlin (New York University Press, 2015), 113.

5 Mintz, "Invisibility," 113. While Mintz writes about invisibility, some scholars and activists opt to use the term *non-apparent disability* for disabilities that aren't visibly discernible. For a more elaborate discussion of non-apparent disability, see Drew Dakessian's entry on the World Institute on Disability's website.

6 Mintz, "Invisibility," 113.

7 These quotations come from the neuropsychological report written for the Minnesota Epilepsy Group dated September 19, 2012 and September 20, 2012.

8 The word *impairment* has a few important connotations in disability studies. Michael Ralph explains how impairment often signifies biological lack, while disability "refers to the process that converts a received deficiency into an obstacle" (107). Just as scholars challenge ideas of normalcy, Ralph reminds us that what constitutes impairment can be critiqued along similar lines. Impairment lies in the

perception—the socially constructed perception—of lack and thereby "endorses the fantasy of a normative human body. Whereas impairment is often treated as an objective fact of the body, many scholars have by now shown how notions of impairment are historically derived, institutionally fixed, and culturally mediated" (108). I tend to use it as signifying lack, with the acknowledgement that this lack is culturally produced.

9 A significant number of research studies look at the power of parental expectations on children, especially in terms of academic achievement. In 2019, Martin Pinquart and Markus Ebeling published a meta-analysis of the impact of parent expectations on their children's academic achievement. The abstract of their article explains how their systematic search identified 169 studies, and their analysis revealed that parental expectations "had an effect over and above the effect of prior achievement" in children. They recommend that parents "communicate positive educational expectations to their children. The transmission of positive expectations to the offspring and the encouragement of academic engagement seem to be more effective in realizing parental expectations than parental behavioural academic involvement such as checking homework and staying in contact with teachers" (463).

10 Chasing a cure for one's disabled child doesn't square with some disability scholars' and activists' ideas of what a good parent would do. From this point of view, my efforts would be best spent advocating for the removal of social barriers that disable my child, not addressing the perceived lack. And yet other disability studies scholars recognize that some surgeries, medications, and prosthetics derived from medical science and technology can relieve pain, increase one's energy to engage in more activities, and generally promote flourishing. As I've mentioned before, Eli Clare's *Brilliant Imperfection: Grappling with Cure* resists the idea that disabled bodies are defective while acknowledging the need to mitigate pain. I agree with Clare, and in this book, I try to illuminate my reflections on what can help or hinder Holden's flourishing.

11 Piepzna-Samarasinha includes her interview with Stacey Milbern in the chapter "Crip Lineages, Crip Futures" of *Care Work*. Milbern articulates the need for disability doulas: "I feel like society not having language to

describe [the transition to disability] or the support it requires speaks to the ableism and isolation people with disabilities face in our lives. Without crip intervention, we are frequently left alone to figure out how to be in our bodyminds and in this ableist world" (240).

12 See Piepzna-Samarasinha, "Crip Lineages," 240.

13 See the chapter "Care Webs: Experiments in Creating Collective Access," where Piepzna-Samarasinha poses a series of provocations designed to generate reflection. Before asking the question that prompted thought for me in the context of this memoir, she also asks: "What does it mean to shift our ideas of access and care (whether it's disability, childcare, economic access, or many more) from an individual chore, an unfortunate cost of having an unfortunate body, to a collective responsibility that's maybe even deeply joyful?" (33). Both these questions generated profound reflection for me regarding not only who I care for and who cares for me but also the attitude and ethic of such care.

CHAPTER ELEVEN

1 Elizabeth Bergmann Loizeaux, *Twentieth-Century Poetry and the Visual Arts* (Cambridge University Press, 2010), 12.

2 Claire Barbetti, *Ekphrastic Medieval Visions: A New Discussion in Interarts Theory* (Palgrave Macmillan, 2011), 11.

3 In my autumn 2014 sabbatical, I researched ekphrasis from a scholarly point of view, despite having practised it as a writer for several years already. I compiled many notes on the books I read, mostly to enrich my creative practice, including Barbara K. Fischer's *Museum Mediations: Reframing Ekphrasis in Contemporary American Poetry*; Elizabeth Bergmann Loizeaux's *Twentieth-Century Poetry and the Visual Arts*; Claire Barbetti's *Ekphrastic Medieval Visions: A New Discussion in Interarts Theory*; Tonya Foster and Kristin Prevallet's edited collection *Third Mind: Creative Writing through Visual Art*; and David Kennedy's *The Ekphrastic Encounter in Contemporary British Poetry and Elsewhere*. Loizeaux is very helpful in tracing the historical changes in the meaning and use of *ekphrasis*, arguing that the Greeks emphasized a particular

kind of description rather than the kind of objects being described (12). Barbetti uses *ekphrasis* as a verb, not a noun, to emphasize the importance of its contemplative aspect: "I believe that the definition needs to take into account the modal agency of *ekphrasis* rather than just its product and recognize the complex processes of perception, memory, translation, interpretation and composition with which it engages" (11). I use the term as both noun and verb, depending on the context, but prefer the rich implications it has for the process of generating insight and new artworks.

4 My inquiry into Katherine of Aragon took root through reading Giles Tremlett's *Catherine of Aragon: Henry's Spanish Queen* and visiting Hampton Court Palace. Katherine piqued my interest because she was an outsider who served her king and new country loyally only to be betrayed by Henry VIII for not producing an heir. As I learned about her education, her series of miscarriages, and the constraints that shaped her political and personal decisions, I marvelled at how much had changed for women in nearly 500 years, and yet how common themes regarding gender-based expectations still keep us bound. A series of epistolary poems contrasts my experiences with Katherine's, and poems from Katherine's point of view use the form of the sonnet. This work can be found in *Creatively Expanding the Premodern: Literary and Historical Afterlives*, a collaboration with Carole Levin, Marguerite A. Tassi, and Julia Griffin.

5 Blackhawk, "Ekphrastic Poetry: Entering and Giving Voice to Works of Art," in *Third Mind: Creative Writing Through Visual Art*, ed. Tonya Foster and Kristin Prevallet (Teachers and Writers Collaborative, 2002), 4.

6 I found this quotation by Monica Prendergast in David Kennedy's *The Ekphrastic Encounter in Contemporary British Poetry and Elsewhere*. Prendergast argues that ekphrastic enquiry is "the representation of research in poetic or other artistic forms. Arts-based enquiry, then, is a way of understanding one kind of experience in terms of another" (12). I appreciated her emphasis on the research and the process of knowledge creation.

7 *Women Collecting Cocoons and Weaving Silk* became the poem "Collecting Cocoons and Weaving Silk," published in *Untrussed* (2016).

This book speaks to the unbinding of relationships, but it also captures the need to make meaning, possibility, and art in the midst of heartbreak. The first poem, "I Wonder," introduces a key thematic element—perspective—both via its classic definition (a way of regarding situations) and its artistic definition (the appearance of things relative to one another as determined by their distance from the viewer). Perspectives pervade the book—the perspective of an outsider in Russia, Italy, and India; the perspective of a viewer of medieval, modern, and contemporary art; the perspective of Wonder Woman—all brought to bear on the dissolution of love and the sustaining force of desire.

CHAPTER TWELVE

1 Alison Kafer, *Feminist, Queer, Crip* (Indiana University Press, 2013), 27.

2 See Kafer, *Feminist, Queer, Crip*, 28.

3 The parent memoirs that I admire most—and that have influenced my writerly decisions in *Silence and Seizure*—have been complex, often expressing two or more difficult-to-reconcile realities at once. Michael Bérubé's *Life as We Know It: A Father, a Family, and an Exceptional Child* is one of those books. In the third chapter, "Sapping the Strength of the State," Bérubé describes the changes his family had to adjust to in the years before and after the birth of his second son, Jamie. He writes: "I had begun to realize, reluctantly, how angry I was with the course my life had taken, not merely because of Jamie's arrival but, instead, because of what it represented: yet another indefinite, prolonged period of stress, another few months or years of waiting to see whether everything would be all right once we were through with X" (97). In the list of stressors, Bérubé includes graduate school, a new job, his oldest son's dangerous asthma, and Jamie's arrival, given the assortment of medical stresses that accompanied his birth with Down syndrome. It felt so refreshing to see this noted, and also to see how "the manual labor of daily maintenance work was salvific both in its demand for immediate presence of mind and in its capacity for deflection and distraction" (99). Like Bérubé noted in his own life, the work of that summer—especially

getting the house ready to sell and acting on the research that I'd done—held a power that helped solidify my reorientation.

4 Kafer, *Feminist, Queer, Crip*, 37.

5 Kafer, *Feminist, Queer, Crip*, 43.

6 An early discussion of teaching sign language to children with acquired epileptic aphasia (LKS) and verbal auditory agnosia was written by Dr. Isabelle Rapin and published in the *Journal of Child Neurology* in 1995.

7 Kafer, *Feminist, Queer, Crip*, 27.

8 Finding out that Holden wasn't a candidate for MST/brain surgery felt far less disappointing than I would have imagined it to be because it took so many months for the surgeon in Chicago to read the MRI and for the professionals at the Minnesota Epilepsy Group to communicate the results to us. By the time I found out, I'd already processed the excitement and dread, and I was just happy to know that I didn't have to worry further about this possibility.

CHAPTER THIRTEEN

1 I wrote down this quotation when I watched the recorded presentation, and the statement was also included in Luther College's media coverage of the event, "Visiting Scholar Rosemarie Garland-Thomson presents 'Building a World that Includes Disability'" by Ava White and Olivia Schmidt.

2 I use statistics about pregnancy after forty only to highlight how unlikely the pregnancy was to occur and carry to term. Although I've seen numbers differ on a few websites, I took this fertility statistic from a webpage on the *Create Fertility* website.

3 This miscarriage statistic comes from an article by Reyhan Harmanci published in the *New York Times*.

4 Rosemarie Garland-Thomson, "The Case for Conserving Disability," *Bioethical Inquiry* (July 2012): 340.

5 In the podcast *The Beagle Has Landed*, Rosemarie Garland-Thomson talks with host Laura Hercher, a genetic counsellor, faculty member, and director of student research at Sarah Lawrence College, about disability rights

in the context of prenatal genetic testing. In the episode, "Difference or Disability?" Garland-Thomson discusses her own identity as a disabled person, the history of disability as an identity group, and the conflict between disabilities and genetic counselling as one of "autonomy and equality, as the right to 'all the information' comes up against the threat of 'eliminating certain classes of persons.'" I found her use of Down syndrome a good example of a "natural human variation" that may confer difference but doesn't preclude a full, joy-filled life, unlike other chromosomal differences that severely limit the life span of an infant.

6 Garland-Thomson, "The Case for Conserving Disability," 353.

7 Whether to have another child after one child is born disabled or develops a disability is a common question in the parent memoirs I've read. In *The Accidental Teacher: Life Lessons from My Silent Son*, Annie Lubliner Lehmann labours over the decision to add to her family, in part due to the intense parenting she carries out for her autistic son, Jonah. Although I found myself troubled by some of Lehmann's assertions, I related to the following passage during my pregnancy with Xavier: "'G-d gives you what you can handle,' was the coined response I often heard when people learned of Jonah's autism. I resented the comment, a platitude meant as an answer for the unexplainable. Yet when I became pregnant, I wanted those words to be true. If I was getting another crack at motherhood, I hoped G-d would see how much we had to handle and cut us some slack" (52).

8 Garland-Thomson, "The Case for Conserving Disability," 353.

CHAPTER FOURTEEN

1 Janice McLaughlin, "Understanding Disabled Families: Replacing Tales of Burden and Resilience with Ties of Interdependency," in *Routledge Handbook of Disability Studies*, 2nd ed., ed. Nick Watson and Simo Vehmas (Taylor & Francis, 2019), 479.

2 McLaughlin, "Understanding Disabled Families," 486.

3 McLaughlin, "Understanding Disabled Families," 481.

4 In Nancy Mairs's memoir, *Waist-High in the World*, she explores, among other rich ideas, what it means to care and be cared for: "I yearn to act out my love in a way that a dancer inscribes abstract movements on the air with hands and feet and torso and head in order to give her private vision public force. I want to *do* love" (79). Mairs describes both the ways others show her love and care and the ways she shows love and care—particularly through deep listening and conversation, because her multiple sclerosis precludes more physical forms. This insight resonated with me, helping me see how my sons, very early in their relationship, created a strong bond based on mutual care, showing their love for each other according to their strengths, abilities, and personalities. Mairs also reinforced for me the truth that care goes both ways, and as I thought about this in regard to Holden, I understood how he needed to be the carer as much as he needed to be cared for to fully flourish.

5 McLaughlin, "Understanding Disabled Families," 483. She continues: "The reality for many disabilities is that medicine is part of life, and the social and political implications of this for disabled families is to ensure that this involvement does not become the key factor in shaping the person's life and identity, or that of those around them, and that medical actors do not become too powerful in dictating the choices and experiences of that person and family (Larson 1998)" (484).

6 I use "survived" deliberately after seeing an adult who had outgrown LKS use it on a discussion board. I think it captures the emotional truth of what it must feel like during the years when the seizure disorder is active.

7 McLaughlin, "Understanding Disabled Families," 483.

8 McLaughlin, "Understanding Disabled Families," 483.

EPILOGUE

1 Many other parents of disabled children who write memoirs mention "Welcome to Holland." I debated using it—was it too cliché? But my decision to reference this piece feels like completing a rite of passage. I appreciate the deep impact that Emily Perl Kingsley's words had on so

many families—how they gave them a framework. For many years, my anger with this piece emerged from its lack of nuance, its implications without explanations. In some ways, this book is my answer to the questions "Welcome to Holland" generated.

2 Rosemarie Garland-Thomson's work became the springboard for my self-designed learning in feminist disability studies and critical disability studies. Her website, which features written work as well as lectures, keynotes, and podcasts, was a rich resource for my initial inquiry.

WORKS CITED

Adams, Rachel. "Disability." *Keywords for Disability Studies*, edited by Rachel Adams, Benjamin Reiss, and David Serlin, 1–11. New York University Press, 2015.

Adams, Rachel. *Raising Henry: A Memoir of Motherhood, Disability, and Discovery*. Reprint edition. Yale University Press, 2014.

Akay, Aynur Pekcanlar, S. Hiz Kurul, H. Ozek, S. Cengizhan, N. Emiroglu, and H. Ellidokuz. "Maternal Reactions to a Child with Epilepsy: Depression, Anxiety, Parental Attitudes and Family Functions." *Epilepsy Research* 95, no. 3 (2011): 213–20. https://doi.org/10.1016/j.eplepsyres.2011.03.020.

Albaradie, Raidah. "Epileptic Encephalopathy Syndromes in Infancy." *Epilepsy in Children – Clinical and Social Aspects*, September 15, 2011. https://doi.org/10.5772/18344.

Alpern, Carol Sober. "Identification and Treatment of Landau-Kleffner Syndrome." *The ASHA Leader Archive* 15, no. 11 (September 2010): 34–35. https://doi.org/10.1044/leader.FTR3.15112010.34.

American College of Obstetricians and Gynecologists. "ACOG Practice Bulletin. Management of Recurrent Pregnancy Loss." *International Journal of Gynaecology and Obstetrics* 78, no. 2 (2002): 179–90. https://doi.org/10.1016/s0020-7292(02)00197-2.

Angelou, Maya. *I Know Why the Caged Bird Sings*. Ballantine Books, 1969.

Atwood, Margaret. *The Journals of Susanna Moodie*. Oxford University Press, 1970.

Baggott, Julianna. *Lizzie Borden in Love: Poems in Women's Voices*. Southern Illinois University Press, 2006.

Barbetti, Claire. *Ekphrastic Medieval Visions: A New Discussion in Interarts Theory*. Palgrave Macmillan, 2011.

Bertram, Edward. "The Relevance of Kindling for Human Epilepsy." Epilepsia 48, suppl. 2 (2007): 65–74. https://doi.org/10.1111/j.1528-1167.2007.01068.x.

Bérubé, Michael. *Life as We Know It: A Father, a Family, and an Exceptional Child.* Vintage, 1998.

Blackhawk, Terry. "Ekphrastic Poetry: Entering and Giving Voice to Works of Art." In *Third Mind: Creative Writing Through Visual Art*, edited by Tonya Foster and Kristin Prevallet, 1–14. Teachers and Writers Collaborative, 2002.

Boutelle, Annie. *Becoming Bone: Poems on the Life of Celia Thaxter (1835–1894)*. University of Arkansas Press, 2005.

Cahalan, Susannah. *Brain on Fire: My Month of Madness*. Simon & Schuster, 2012.

Campbell, Fiona Kumari. "Ability." In *Keywords for Disability Studies*, edited by Rachel Adams, Benjamin Reiss, and David Serlin, 12–14. New York University Press, 2015.

Centers for Disease Control and Prevention. "Epilepsy." https://www.cdc.gov/epilepsy/first-aid-for-seizures/index.html. Accessed January 8, 2025.

Chapieski, Lynn, V. Brewer, K. Evankovich, K. Culhane Shelburne, K. Zelman, and A. Alexander. "Adaptive Functioning in Children with Seizures: Impact of Maternal Anxiety about Epilepsy." *Epilepsy & Behavior* 7, no. 2 (2005): 246–52. https://doi.org/10.1016/j.yebeh.2005.05.002.

Children and Adults with Attention-Deficit/Hyperactivity Disorder (CHADD). "Understanding ADHD." chadd.org/understanding-adhd. Accessed November 24, 2024.

Clare, Eli. *Brilliant Imperfection: Grappling with Cure*. Duke University Press, 2017.

Cohen, Jon. *Coming to Term: Uncovering the Truth about Miscarriage*. Rutgers University Press, 2007.

Create Fertility. "Your Chances of Getting Pregnant at 40 with and without IVF." https://www.createfertility.co.uk/blog. Accessed December 17, 2024.

Dakessian, Drew. "Non-Apparent Disabilities: When Your Disability Is Not Visible." World Institute on Disability. https://www.wid.org. Accessed December 10, 2024.

DeSalvo, Louise. *Writing as a Way of Healing: How Telling Our Stories Transforms Our Lives*. Beacon Press, 2000.

Eisenmenger, Ashley. "Ableism 101." *Access Living*, December 12, 2019, https://www.accessliving.org/newsroom/blog/ableism-101/. Accessed November 8, 2024.

Epilepsy Foundation. "Complications and Risks." https://www.epilepsy.com/complications-risks. Accessed November 18, 2024.

Epilepsy Foundation. "Seizure Triggers." https://www.epilepsy.com. Accessed November 12, 2024.

Epilepsy Foundation. "Understanding Epilepsy." https://www.epilepsy.com. Accessed November 12, 2024.

Epilepsy Foundation. "What is Epilepsy? / Types of Seizures." https://www.epilepsy.com. Accessed November 12, 2024.

Erevelles, Nirmala. *Disability and Difference in Global Contexts: Enabling a Transformative Body Politic*. Palgrave Macmillan, 2016.

Erevelles, Nirmala, and Alison Kafer. "Committed Critique: An Interview with Nirmala Erevelles." *Deaf and Disability Studies: Interdisciplinary Perspectives*, edited by Susan Burch and Alison Kafer, 204–21. Gallaudet University Press, 2010.

Fischer, Barbara K. *Museum Mediations: Reframing Ekphrasis in Contemporary American Poetry*. Routledge, 2006.

Foster, Tonya, and Kristin Prevallet, eds. *Third Mind: Creative Writing through Visual Art*. Teachers and Writers Collaborative, 2002.

Gabbard, Chris. *A Life Beyond Reason: A Father's Memoir*. Beacon Press, 2019.

Garland-Thomson, Rosemarie. "Becoming Disabled." *New York Times*, August 19, 2016, Sunday Opinion.

Garland-Thomson, Rosemarie. "The Case for Conserving Disability." *Bioethical Inquiry*, July (2012): 339–55.

Garland-Thomson, Rosemarie. "Feminist Disability Studies." *Signs: Journal of Women in Culture and Society* 30, no. 2 (2005): 1557–87.

Garland-Thomson, Rosemarie. "Rosemarie Garland-Thomson." https://rosemariegarlandthomson.com. Accessed November 2021.

Grady, Denise. "Doctors Put Hope in Thin Wires to Ease the Clutches of Epilepsy." *New York Times*, May 24, 2004. https://www.nytimes.com/2004/05/24/us/doctors-put-hope-in-thin-wires-to-ease-the-clutches-of-epilepsy.html.

Grote, Christopher L., Patricia Van Slyke, and Jo-Ann B. Hoeppner. "Language Outcome Following Multiple Subpial Transection for Landau-Kleffner Syndrome." *Brain* 122, no. 3 (March 1999): 561–66.

Gutkind, Lee, ed. *Keep It Real: Everything You Need to Know About Researching and Writing Creative Nonfiction*. W.W. Norton, 2008.

Harmanci, Reyhan. "The Truth About Pregnancy Over 40." *The New York Times*, April 15, 2020. Updated March 29, 2022. https://www.nytimes.com/2020/04/15/parenting/pregnancy/baby-after-40.html.

Hercher, Laura. "Difference or Disability? with Rosemarie Garland-Thomson." *The Beagle Has Landed*, October 27, 2020, https://www.beaglelanded.com/podcasts. Accessed December 11, 2024.

Holmes, Gregory L. "Epilepsy Syndromes." Epilepsy Foundation, January 1, 2008. https://www.epilepsy.com/what-is-epilepsy/syndromes. Accessed November 27, 2024.

Hopper, Kate. *Use Your Words: A Writing Guide for Mothers*. Viva Editions, 2012.

Horton, Jillian. *We Are All Perfectly Fine: A Memoir of Love, Medicine, and Healing*. HarperCollins, 2021.

Hurston, Zora Neale. *Dust Tracks on the Road: An Autobiography*. HarperPerennial, 1942.

Johns Hopkins Medicine. "Diagnosing Seizures and Epilepsy." https://www.hopkinsmedicine.org. Accessed December 11, 2024.

Jones, Chloe, and Colin Reilly. "Parental Anxiety in Childhood Epilepsy: A Systematic Review." *Epilepsia* 57, no. 4 (2016): 529–37. https://doi.org/10.1111/epi.13326.

Joshi, Charuta. "Developmental/Epileptic Encephalopathy with Spike Wave Activation in Sleep (DEE-SWAS)." *Epilepsy Foundation*, https://www.epilepsy.com/what-is-epilepsy/syndromes/dee-swas. Accessed October 9, 2025.

Kafer, Alison. *Feminist, Queer, Crip*. Indiana University Press, 2013.

Kennedy, David. *The Ekphrastic Encounter in Contemporary British Poetry and Elsewhere*. Routledge, 2012.

Khakpour, Porochista. *Sick: A Memoir*. HarperCollins, 2018.

Kingsley, Emily Perl. "Welcome to Holland." https://emilyperlkingsley.com. Accessed January 8, 2025.

Kittay, Eva. *Learning from My Daughter: The Value and Care of Disabled Minds*. Oxford University Press, 2019.

Kleege, Georgina. *Blind Rage: Letters to Helen Keller*. Gallaudet University Press, 2006.

Kleege, Georgina. *Sight Unseen*. Yale University Press, 1999.

Kooser, Ted. "Lying for the Sake of Making Poems." *After Confession: Poetry as Autobiography,* edited by Kate Sontag and David Graham, 158–61. Graywolf Press, 2001.

Kuusisto, Stephen. *Planet of the Blind.* Delta Press, 1998.

Lanier, Heather. *Raising a Rare Girl: A Memoir.* Penguin Press, 2020.

Lauren, Jillian. *Everything You Ever Wanted: A Memoir*. Plume Press, 2015.

Lehmann, Annie Lubliner. *The Accidental Teacher: Life Lessons from My Silent Son*. University of Michigan Press, 2009.

Limburg, Joanne. *Letters to My Weird Sisters: On Autism and Feminism.* Atlantic Books, 2021.

Loizeaux, Elizabeth Bergmann. *Twentieth century Poetry and the Visual Arts.* Cambridge University Press, 2010.

Lorde, Audre. *The Cancer Journals*. Penguin, 1980.

Lorde, Audre. *Zami: A New Spelling of My Name: A Biomythography.* Crossing Press, 1982.

Love, Heather. "Stigma." *Keywords for Disability Studies*, edited by Rachel Adams, Benjamin Reiss, and David Serlin, 173–76. New York University Press, 2015.

Lv, R., L. Wu, L. Jin, Q. Lu, M. Wang, Y. Qu, and H. Liu. "Depression, Anxiety and Quality of Life in Parents of Children with Epilepsy." *Acta Neurologica Scandinavica* 120 (2009): 335–41. https://doi.org/10.1111/j.1600-0404.2009.01184.x.

Mairs, Nancy. *Waist-High in the World: A Life Among the Nondisabled*. Beacon Press, 1996.

Manokaran, Ranjith Kumar, Suvasini Sharma, and Rajesh Ramachandrannair. "The 2022 International League Against Epilepsy Classification and Definition of Childhood Epilepsy Syndromes: An Update for Pediatricians." *Indian Pediatrics* 61, no. 2 (2024): 179–83. https://pubmed.ncbi.nlm.nih.gov/38321731/. Accessed December 4, 2024.

Mayo Clinic. "Divalproex sodium." https://www.mayoclinic.org/drugs. Accessed November 18, 2024.

Mayo Clinic. "Epilepsy / causes." https://www.mayoclinic.org/diseasesconditions/epilepsy/symptoms-causes/syc-20350093. Accessed January 8, 2025.

Mayo Clinic. "Seizures." https://www.mayoclinic.org/diseases/conditions/seizure/symptoms-causes/syc-20365711. Accessed November 10, 2024.

McLaughlin, Janice. "Understanding Disabled Families: Replacing Tales of Burden and Resilience with Ties of Interdependency." *Routledge Handbook of Disability Studies*, 2nd ed., edited by Nick Watson and Simo Vehmas, 479–91. Taylor & Francis, 2019.

Miller, Brenda, and Suzanne Paola. *Tell It Slant: Writing and Shaping Creative Nonfiction*. McGraw Hill, 2004.

Mintz, Susannah B. "Invisibility." *Keywords for Disability Studies*, edited by Rachel Adams, Benjamin Reiss, and David Serlin, 113–14. New York University Press, 2015.

Mirriam-Goldberg, Caryn. "Dragonflies and Inky Blackness: Raising a Child with Asperger's Syndrome." *My Baby Rides the Short Bus: The Unabashedly Human Experience of Raising Kids with Disabilities*, edited by Yantra Bertelli, Jennifer Silverman, and Sarah Talbot, 242–52. PM Press, 2009.

The Miscarriage Association. "Missed Miscarriage." *Miscarriage Association.* https://www.miscarriageassociation.org.uk. Accessed November 15, 2024.

Morales, Aurora Levins. *Kindling: Writings on the Body*. Palabrera, 2013.

Murkoff, Heidi E., and Arlene Eisenberg. *What to Expect When You're Expecting*. 3rd ed. Workman Publishing Company, 2002.

Nuñez, Juan Abel. Personal correspondence, February 17, 2019.

Pereira-Sanchez, Victor, and Francisco X. Castellanos. "Neuroimaging in Attention Deficit/Hyperactivity Disorder." *Current Opinion in Psychiatry* 34, no. 2 (2021), 105–111. https://doi.org/10.1097/YCO.0000000000000669.

Perl, Sondra, and Mimi Schwartz. *Writing True: The Art and Craft of Creative Nonfiction*. 2nd edition. Wadsworth Cengage Learning, 2014.

Piepmeier, Alison. "Saints, Sages, and Victims: Endorsement of and Resistance to Cultural Stereotypes in Memoirs by Parents of Children with Disabilities." *Disability Studies Quarterly* 32, no. 1 (2012).

Piepzna-Samarasinha, Leah Lakshmi. *Care Work: Dreaming Disability Justice*. Arsenal Pulp Press, 2021.

Pinquart, Martin, and Markus Ebeling. "Parental Educational Expectations and Academic Achievement in Children and Adolescents—a Meta-analysis." *Educational Psychology Review* 32, no. 2 (2020): 463–80. https://doi.org/10.1007/s10648-019-09506-z.

Pratt, Sara. "Neuropsychological Report." Minnesota Epilepsy Group. Sept. 19–20, 2012.

Quinn, Hannah, and Rebecca-Eli Long. "Consent-as-Method: Capacity to Consent of Cognitively Disabled People and Research Ethics Review." *Canadian Journal of Disability Studies* 13, no. 1 (April 2024).

Ralph, Michael. "Impairment." *Keywords for Disability Studies*, edited by Rachel Adams, Benjamin Reiss, and David Serlin, 107–8. New York University Press, 2015.

Rapin, Isabelle. "Acquired Aphasia in Children." *Journal of Child Neurology* 10 (1995): 267–70.

Rapp, Emily. *The Still Point of a Turning World*. Penguin, 2013.

Reiheld, Alison. "The Event That Was Nothing: Miscarriage as a Liminal Event." *Journal of Social Philosophy* 46, no. 1 (2015): 9–26.

Rex, Brian T. Personal correspondence. May–September 2012.

Richardson, Laurel. "Writing: A Method of Inquiry." *Handbook of Qualitative Research.* 2nd ed., edited by Norman K. Denzin and Yvonna S. Lincoln, 923–48. Sage Publications, 2000.

Riviello, James J., Jr., and Stavros Hadjiloizou. "The Landau-Kleffner Syndrome and Epilepsy with Continuous Spike-Waves During Sleep." *Behavioral Aspects of Epilepsy: Principles and Practice*, edited by Steven C. Schachter, Gregory L. Holmes, and Dorothée G.A. Kasteleijn-Nolst Trenité, 377–82. Demos Medical Publishing, 2007.

Roripaugh, Lee Ann. *Year of the Snake.* Southern Illinois University Press, 2004.

Sands, Tristan T., and Gelinas, Jennifer N. "Epilepsy and Encephalopathy." *Pediatric Neurology* 150 (2024): 24–31.

Savarese, Ralph James. "Cognition." *Keywords for Disability Studies*, edited by Rachel Adams, Benjamin Reiss, and David Serlin, 40–42. New York University Press, 2015.

Silverman, Amy. *My Heart Can't Even Believe It.* Woodbine House, 2016.

Smith, Michael C., and Thomas J. Hoeppner. "Epileptic Encephalopathy of Late Childhood." *Journal of Clinical Neurophysiology* 20, no. 6 (2003): 462–72.

Solomon, Andrew. *Far from the Tree: Parents, Children and the Search for Identity.* Scribner Classics, 2014.

Stewart-Nuñez, Christine. *Bluewords Greening.* Terrapin Books, 2016.

Stewart-Nuñez, Christine. *Chrysopoeia: Essays of Language, Love, and Place.* Stephen F. Austin University Press, 2022.

Stewart-Nuñez, Christine. "Katherine of Aragon." *Creatively Expanding the Premodern: Historical and Literary Afterlives*, with Carole Levin, Marguerite A. Tassi, Christine Stewart-Nuñez, and Julia Griffin. Routledge, 2026.

Stewart-Nuñez, Christine. *Keeping Them Alive.* WordTech Editions, 2011.

Stewart-Nuñez, Christine. *The Love of Unreal Things.* Finishing Line Press, 2005.

Stewart-Nuñez, Christine. *The Poet & The Architect.* Terrapin Books, 2021.

Stewart-Nuñez, Christine. *Untrussed: Poems.* New Mexico University Press, 2016.

Suglani, Lalitaa. *High-Functioning Anxiety: A Five-Step Guide to Calming the Inner Panic and Thriving, Kindle edition*. Hay House, 2024.

Szuhany, Kristin, and Naomi Simon. "Anxiety Disorders: A Review." *JAMA* 328, no. 24 (2022): 2431–45. https://doi.org/10.1001/jama.2022.22744.

Titchkosky, Tanya. "Normal." *Keywords for Disability Studies*, edited by Rachel Adams, Benjamin Reiss, and David Serlin, 130–32. New York University Press, 2015.

Tschumi, Bernard. *Architecture and Disjunction*. MIT Press, 1996.

White, Ava, and Olivia Schmidt. "Visiting Scholar Rosemarie Garland-Thomson Presents 'Building a World That Includes Disability.'" *Chips*. Luther College, May 8, 2002. https://lutherchips.com/9683/news/visiting-scholar-rosemarie-garland-thomson-presents-building-a-world-that-includes-disability/. Accessed December 17, 2024.

World Health Organization. "Epilepsy." World Health Organization, February 7, 2024. https://www.who.int/news-room/fact-sheets/detail/epilepsy. Accessed November 10, 2024.

Published by Wilfrid Laurier University Press

BOOKS IN THE LIFE WRITING SERIES

Haven't Any News: Ruby's Letters from the Fifties edited by Edna Staebler with an afterword by Marlene Kadar • 1995 • x + 172 pp. • ISBN 978-0-88920-248-1

"I Want to Join Your Club": Letters from Rural Children, 1900–1920 edited by Norah L. Lewis with a preface by Neil Sutherland • 1996 • xii + 250 pp. • 30 b&w photos • ISBN 978-0-88920-260-3

And Peace Never Came by Elisabeth M. Raab with historical notes by Marlene Kadar • 1996 • x + 196 pp. • 12 b&w photos, 1 map • ISBN 978-0-88920-292-4

Dear Editor and Friends: Letters from Rural Women of the North-West, 1900–1920 edited by Norah L. Lewis • 1998 • xvi + 166 pp. • 20 b&w photos • ISBN 978-0-88920-287-0

The Surprise of My Life: An Autobiography by Claire Drainie Taylor with a foreword by Marlene Kadar • 1998 • xii + 268 pp. • 8 colour photos, 92 b&w photos • ISBN 978-0-88920-302-0

BOOKS IN THE LIFE WRITING SERIES

Memoirs from Away: A New Found Land Girlhood by Helen M. Buss / Margaret Clarke • 1998 • xvi + 154 pp. • ISBN 978-0-88920-350-1

The Life and Letters of Annie Leake Tuttle: Working for the Best by Marilyn Färdig Whiteley • 1999 • xviii + 150 pp. • ISBN 978-0-88920-330-3

Marian Engel's Notebooks: "Ah, mon cahier, écoute..." edited by Christl Verduyn • 1999 • viii + 576 pp. • ISBN 978-0-88920-349-5

Be Good, Sweet Maid: The Trials of Dorothy Joudrie by Audrey Andrews • 1999 • vi + 276 pp. • ISBN 978-0-88920-334-1

Working in Women's Archives: Researching Women's Private Literature and Archival Documents edited by Helen M. Buss and Marlene Kadar • 2001 • vi + 120 pp. • ISBN 978-0-88920-341-9

Repossessing the World: Reading Memoirs by Contemporary Women by Helen M. Buss • 2002 • xxvi + 206 pp. • ISBN 978-0-88920-409-6

Chasing the Comet: A Scottish-Canadian Life by Patricia Koretchuk • 2002 • xx + 244 pp. • ISBN 978-0-88920-407-2

The Queen of Peace Room by Magie Dominic • 2002 • xiv + 114 pp. • ISBN 978-0-88920-417-1

China Diary: The Life of Mary Austin Endicott by Shirley Jane Endicott • 2002 • xvi + 254 pp. • ISBN 978-0-88920-412-6

The Curtain: Witness and Memory in Wartime Holland by Henry G. Schogt • 2003 • xii + 132 pp. • ISBN 978-0-88920-396-9

Teaching Places by Audrey J. Whitson • 2003 • xiv + 182 pp. • 9 colour photos • ISBN 978-0-88920-425-6

Through the Hitler Line: Memoirs of an Infantry Chaplain by Laurence F. Wilmot, M.C. • 2003 • xvi + 152 pp. • ISBN 978-0-88920-448-5

Where I Come From by Vijay Agnew • 2003 • xiv + 298 pp. • ISBN 978-0-88920-414-0

The Water Lily Pond: A Village Girl's Journey in Maoist China by Han Z. Li • 2004 • x + 254 pp. • ISBN 978-0-88920-431-7

The Life Writings of Mary Baker McQuesten: Victorian Matriarch edited by Mary J. Anderson • 2004 • xxii + 338 pp. • ISBN 978-0-88920-437-9

Seven Eggs Today: The Diaries of Mary Armstrong, 1859 and 1869 edited by Jackson W. Armstrong • 2004 • xvi + 228 pp. • ISBN 978-0-55458-439-0

Incorrigible by Velma Demerson • 2004 • vi + 178 pp. • ISBN 978-0-88920-444-7

Love and War in London: A Woman's Diary 1939–1942 by Olivia Cockett; edited by Robert W. Malcolmson • 2005 • xvi + 208 pp. • ISBN 978-0-88920-458-4

Auto/biography in Canada: Critical Directions edited by Julie Rak • 2005 • viii + 264 pp. • ISBN 978-0-88920-478-2

Tracing the Autobiographical edited by Marlene Kadar, Linda Warley, Jeanne Perreault, and Susanna Egan • 2005 • viii + 280 pp. • ISBN 978-0-88920-476-8

Must Write: Edna Staebler's Diaries edited by Christl Verduyn • 2005 • viii + 304 pp. • ISBN 978-0-88920-481-2

Pursuing Giraffe: A 1950s Adventure by Anne Innis Dagg • 2006 • xvi + 284 pp. • 46 b&w photos, 2 maps • ISBN 978-0-88920-463-8

Food That Really Schmecks by Edna Staebler • 2007 • xxiv + 334 pp. • ISBN 978-0-88920-521-5

163256: A Memoir of Resistance by Michael Englishman • 2007 • xvi + 112 pp. • 14 b&w photos • ISBN 978-1-55458-009-5

The Wartime Letters of Leslie and Cecil Frost, 1915–1919 edited by R.B. Fleming • 2007 • xxxvi + 384 pp. • 49 b&w photos, 5 maps • ISBN 978-1-55458-470-3

Johanna Krause Twice Persecuted: Surviving in Nazi Germany and Communist East Germany by Carolyn Gammon and Christiane Hemker • 2007 • x + 170 pp. • 58 b&w photos, 2 maps • ISBN 978-1-55458-006-4

Watermelon Syrup: A Novel by Annie Jacobsen with Jane Finlay-Young and Di Brandt • 2007 • x + 268 pp. • ISBN 978-1-55458-005-7

Broad Is the Way: Stories from Mayerthorpe by Margaret Norquay • 2008 • x + 106 pp. • 6 b&w photos • ISBN 978-1-55458-020-0

Becoming My Mother's Daughter: A Story of Survival and Renewal by Erika Gottlieb • 2008 • x + 178 pp. • 53 colour and b&w illus. • ISBN 978-1-55458-030-9

Leaving Fundamentalism: Personal Stories edited by G. Elijah Dann • 2008 • xii + 234 pp. • ISBN 978-1-55458-026-2

Bearing Witness: Living with Ovarian Cancer edited by Kathryn Carter and Lauri Elit • 2009 • viii + 94 pp. • ISBN 978-1-55458-055-2

Dead Woman Pickney: A Memoir of Childhood in Jamaica by Yvonne Shorter Brown • 2010 • viii + 202 pp. • ISBN 978-1-55458-189-4

BOOKS IN THE LIFE WRITING SERIES

I Have a Story to Tell You by Seemah C. Berson • 2010 • xx + 288 pp. • 24 b&w photos • ISBN 978-1-55458-219-8

We All Giggled: A Bourgeois Family Memoir by Thomas O. Hueglin • 2010 • xiv + 232 pp. • 20 b&w photos • ISBN 978-1-55458-262-4

Just a Larger Family: Letters of Marie Williamson from the Canadian Home Front, 1940–1944 edited by Mary F. Williamson and Tom Sharp • 2011 • xxiv + 378 pp. • 16 b&w photos • ISBN 978-1-55458-323-2

Burdens of Proof: Faith, Doubt, and Identity in Autobiography by Susanna Egan • 2011 • x + 200 pp. • ISBN 978-1-55458-333-1

Accident of Fate: A Personal Account 1938–1945 by Imre Rochlitz with Joseph Rochlitz • 2011 • xiv + 226 pp. • 50 b&w photos, 5 maps • ISBN 978-1-55458-267-9

The Green Sofa by Natascha Würzbach, translated by Raleigh Whitinger • 2012 • xiv + 240 pp. • 5 b&w photos • ISBN 978-1-55458-334-8

Unheard Of: Memoirs of a Canadian Composer by John Beckwith • 2012 • x + 394 pp. • 74 b&w illus., 8 musical examples • ISBN 978-1-55458-358-4

Borrowed Tongues: Life Writing, Migration, and Translation by Eva C. Karpinski • 2012 • viii + 274 pp. • ISBN 978-1-55458-357-7

Basements and Attics, Closets and Cyberspace: Explorations in Canadian Women's Archives edited by Linda M. Morra and Jessica Schagerl • 2012 • x + 338 pp. • ISBN 978-1-77112-328-0

The Memory of Water by Allen Smutylo • 2013 • x + 262 pp. • 65 colour illus. • ISBN 978-1-55458-842-8

The Unwritten Diary of Israel Unger, Revised Edition by Carolyn Gammon and Israel Unger • 2013 • x + 230 pp. • 90 b&w illus. • ISBN 978-1-77112-011-1

Boom!: Manufacturing Memoir for the Popular Market by Julie Rak • 2013 • viii + 250 pp. • 7 b&w illus. • ISBN 978-1-55458-939-5

Motherlode: A Mosaic of Dutch Wartime Experience by Carolyne Van Der Meer • 2014 • xiv + 132 pp. • 6 b&w illus. • ISBN 978-1-77112-005-0

Not the Whole Story: Challenging the Single Mother Narrative edited by Lea Caragata and Judit Alcalde • 2014 • x + 222 pp. • ISBN 978-1-55458-624-0

Street Angel by Magie Dominic • 2014 • viii + 154 pp. • ISBN 978-1-77112-026-5

BOOKS IN THE LIFE WRITING SERIES

In the Unlikeliest of Places: How Nachman Libeskind Survived the Nazis, Gulags, and Soviet Communism by Annette Libeskind Berkovits with a foreword by Daniel Libeskind • 2014 • xiv + 282 pp. • 6 colour illus. • ISBN 978-1-77112-066-1

Kinds of Winter: Four Solo Journeys by Dogteam in Canada's Northwest Territories by Dave Olesen • 2014 • xii + 256 pp. • 17 b&w illus., 6 maps • ISBN 978-1-77112-131-6

Working Memory: Women and Work in World War II edited by Marlene Kadar and Jeanne Perreault • 2015 • viii + 246 pp. • 46 b&w and colour illus. • ISBN 978-1-77112-035-7

Wait Time: A Memoir of Cancer by Kenneth Sherman • 2016 • xiv + 138 pp. • ISBN 978-1-77112-188-0

Canadian Graphic: Picturing Life Narratives edited by Candida Rifkind and Linda Warley • 2016 • viii + 310 pp. • 59 colour and b&w illus. • ISBN 978-1-77112-179-8

Travels and Identities: Elizabeth and Adam Shortt in Europe, 1911 edited by Peter E. Paul Dembski • 2017 • xxii + 272 pp. • 9 b&w illus. • ISBN 978-1-77112-225-2

Bird-Bent Grass: A Memoir, in Pieces by Kathleen Venema • 2018 • viii + 346 pp. • ISBN 978-1-77112-290-0

My Basilian Priesthood, 1961 to 1967 by Michael Quealey with an afterword by Arthur Haberman and Jan Rehner • 2019 • viii + 222 pp. • ISBN 978-1-77112-242-9

What the Oceans Remember: Searching for Belonging and Home by Sonja Boon • 2019 • xvi + 320 pp. • 8 b&w illus. • ISBN 978-1-77112-553-6

Rough and Plenty: A Memorial by Raymond A. Rogers • 2020 • x + 316 pp. • 9 b&w photos • ISBN 978-1-77112-436-2

Limelight: Canadian Women and the Rise of Celebrity Autobiography by Katja Lee • 2020 • viii + 360 pp. • 6 colour images • ISBN 978-1-77112-429-4

Prison Life Writing: Conversion and the Literary Roots of the U.S. Prison System by Simon Rolston • 2021 • x + 316 pp. • ISBN 978-1-77112-517-8

Scratching River by Michelle Porter • 2022 • xiv + 168 pp. • ISBN 978-1-77112-544-4

BOOKS IN THE LIFE WRITING SERIES

Dead Woman Pickney: A Memoir of Childhood in Jamaica, Second Edition by Yvonne Shorter Brown with a foreword by Sonja Boon • 2022 • xxvi + 318 pp. • 9 b&w images • ISBN 978-1-77112-547-5

Erasing Frankenstein: Remaking the Monster, A Public Humanities Prison Arts Project edited by Elizabeth Effinger • 2024 • x + 344 pp. • 178 colour images • ISBN 978-1-77112-618-2

Unequivocal Magic: Sarah Bernhardt and the Journey of a Portrait by Alex Bertram • 2026 • xviii + 198 pp. • 19 b&w images • ISBN 978-1-77112-718-9

Silence and Seizure by Christine Stewart-Nuñez • 2026 • xiv + 286 pp. • ISBN 978-1-77112-733-2